Hèla Ben Jmaà
Rania Hammami
Nesrine Ghorbel

Acute mitral insufficiency after percutaneous commissurotomy

Hèla Ben Jmaà
Rania Hammami
Nesrine Ghorbel

Acute mitral insufficiency after percutaneous commissurotomy

ScienciaScripts

Imprint
Any brand names and product names mentioned in this book are subject to trademark, brand or patent protection and are trademarks or registered trademarks of their respective holders. The use of brand names, product names, common names, trade names, product descriptions etc. even without a particular marking in this work is in no way to be construed to mean that such names may be regarded as unrestricted in respect of trademark and brand protection legislation and could thus be used by anyone.

Cover image: www.ingimage.com

This book is a translation from the original published under ISBN 978-620-6-71774-4.

Publisher:
Sciencia Scripts
is a trademark of
Dodo Books Indian Ocean Ltd. and OmniScriptum S.R.L publishing group

120 High Road, East Finchley, London, N2 9ED, United Kingdom
Str. Armeneasca 28/1, office 1, Chisinau MD-2012, Republic of Moldova, Europe
Printed at: see last page
ISBN: 978-620-8-25343-1

Acute mitral insufficiency after percutaneous commissurotomy

I- Introduction :

Acute rheumatic fever (ARF) is still a common disease in developing countries.

In Tunisia, the incidence of AAR has fallen steadily. This epidemiological improvement is linked to the national programme to combat AAR, which has long been regarded as a major public health problem.

Rheumatic valve disease, mainly mitral stenosis, is a major problem in France.

Percutaneous mitral commissurotomy is the treatment of choice for pure narrowing (MR). It allows the obstacle to be removed with a lower morbidity and mortality and less harm than surgical techniques.

However, it can be complicated by acute mitral insufficiency (MI) requiring emergency surgery.

The Wilkins score is a semi-quantitative echocardiographic score proposed by Wilkins et al [1]. It consists of quantifying from 1 to 4 the severity of the alteration of the four following parameters:

- Valve mobility (Wilkins 1) is studied on the left paraspinal long axis (PSGGA) and apical 4-cavity sections. It is graded from 1 to 4.

- The subvalvular apparatus (SVA) (Wilkins 2) is studied mainly on the apical 2-cavity section but also on the PSGGA section. It is graded from 1 to 4.

- Valvular thickening (Wilkins 3): on PSGGA and left parasternal short axis (PSGPA) sections. It is graded from 1 to 4.

- Valvular calcification (Wilkins 4): mainly on PSGGA and PSGPA sections. It is graded from 1 to 4.

The final score is the sum of the individual scores and varies from 4 to 16.

The steps in the dilation procedure are (Figure 1):

-        Right and left heart catheterisation

-        Trans-septal catheterisation: this is a key stage which determines whether the procedure can continue, and carries a risk of complications, particularly haemopericardial. It is performed using the Brockenbrough needle.

This step of crossing the atrial septum is followed by an injection of 1 mg/Kg of heparin, not to exceed 50 mg.

- A guide is inserted into the Mullins sheath via the right femoral vein, with a very flexible end that coils in the left atrium.

- The sheath is removed and the 14 F dilator is fitted to the guide, dilating the femoral puncture site and the septum.

- Once the dilator has been removed and the tube inserted into the central lumen of the balloon catheter and locked in place, the catheter is advanced over the guide and across the septum.

- When the tip of the balloon is close to the roof of the left atrium, withdraw the tube by 2 to 3 cm.

- Simultaneous removal of the tube and guide and partial inflation of the balloon

- Once the J guide is in place, the mitral valve is crossed and partial inflation is performed to confirm its correct position by the appearance of the commissural indentations.

- Complete inflation by manual injection followed by immediate deflation, lasting on average 5 to 6 seconds, with hypotension and ventricular extra-systole per-inflation.

- Haemodynamic monitoring of the result.

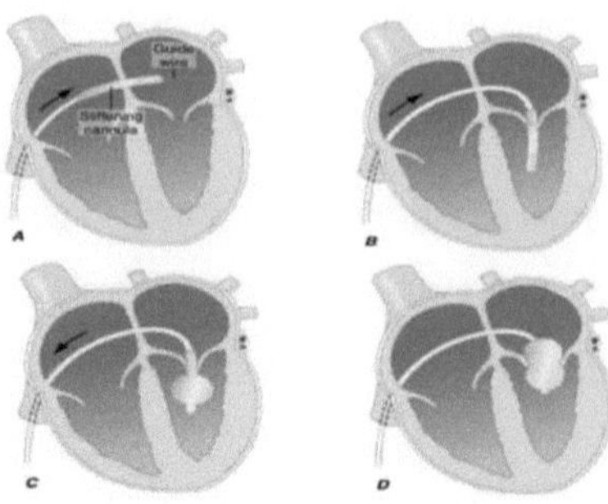

Figure 1: Schematic of percutaneous transvenous valvuloplasty [2].

The ASA score must be determined. This is a score used to express a patient's pre-operative state of health. It is used to assess anaesthetic risk and to obtain a predictive parameter for perioperative mortality and morbidity [3].

EuroSCORE II, or the European System for Cardiac Operative Risk Evaluation, was developed by the European Association of CardioThoracic Surgery. It is a single score for all types of cardiac surgery [4, 5, 6].

The operation is performed on bypass graft with the aorta clamped. The purpose of bypass surgery, which is an artificial heart-lung machine, is to temporarily replace the pumping and haematosis functions performed by the heart and lung respectively. This makes it possible to open the heart chambers and perform surgery on a stopped, bloodless heart [7].

II- Epidemiological characteristics of patients :

1- Age :

The average age of PMCD in Tunisia is young, which is explained by the predominance of rheumatic fever [8]. The average age in the literature is older [9, 10].

In the series by Ruiz et al [9], the mean age was 49, and in the series by Lung et al [10], the mean age was 45.

2- Gender :

The predominance of female patients has been found in various series around the world [11]. This is related to the fact that rheumatic fever is the main aetiology and that RAA predominates in female patients.

III- Immediate results of the procedure :

1- Procedural success:

The success of the percutaneous commissurotomy procedure is defined by some authors as the achievement of a mitral surface area greater than 1.5 cm^2 in the absence of mitral insufficiency greater than grade II [12].

Other authors define the success of the procedure by a gain in surface area of 50% compared with the initial surface area, or a mitral surface area greater than 1 cm2 /m2 of body surface area. Others define success as the opening of at least one commissure.

The procedural success rate varies from 75 to 98% depending on the series [13, 14, 15, 16].

2- Immediate complications:

Possible complications during this procedure are :

- Procedural failure: varies between 1 and 15% depending on the series [17].

- Death: the mortality rate for percutaneous mitral dilation varies from 0.5 to 4% [18]. The main cause of death is tamponade due to perforation of the LV.

- Haemopericardium and tamponade: This is the most serious complication. Its incidence varies between 0 and 2% depending on the series [19]. It often occurs during the trans-septal puncture stage.

- Systemic embolisms: In the literature, embolic accidents occur with a frequency varying from 0 to 5% [18, 20, 21, 29]. These are mainly cerebrovascular accidents (CVA) caused either by migration of a left intra-atrial thrombus, rupture of a poorly purged balloon or migration of a clot formed on the balloon.

- Acute mitral insufficiency: This is the most frequent complication in SCPD. This study focuses on this complication.

IV- Post-procedural acute mitral insufficiency :

It may appear de novo, or it may result from the aggravation of a pre-existing MI.

1- Incidence :

While minimal (grade I) or moderate (grade II) MI is usual after DMPC, severe MI (grade III or IV) is rare and constitutes a genuine complication.

MI is moderate in 50% of cases, while an increase in degree is found in 1/3 of cases without any haemodynamic deterioration being observed [22].

Indeed, Block and Palacios [23] showed a reduction in the severity of MI in 53% of cases in patients who developed mitral insufficiency after valvuloplasty. They explain this phenomenon by the reversible stretching of mitral tissue during and after valvuloplasty and its healing, the healing of commissural tears reaching the annulus, and the reversible malfunction of the papillary muscles secondary to the traumatic irritation of the balloon.

A MI was created in 21% of cases in the series by Hernandez et al [24], in 24% of cases in the series by Lung et al [25], and in 21.5% of cases in the series by Ben Farhat et al [26]. In the series by Pathan et al [27], 5.5% of the population had an MI > grade 3 post DMPC. Lung et al [28] showed in a review of all the DMPC series between 1986 and 2002 that the procedural failure rate had decreased significantly, but that the rate of MI remained stable.

The incidence of severe MI varies from 1 to 10% in most series [12, 18,

27]. It depends on the experience of the team. It has been reduced by training in the technique, the use of appropriately sized balloons, and the selection of candidates by pre-procedural ultrasound analysis of valve anatomy.

Literature data are summarised in Table I.

Table I: Incidence of acute severe MI in different series in the literature.

Author (year)	Number of procedures	Severe MI
Vahanian (1991) [29]	600	3.8%
Alfonso (1993) [30]	288	7%
Chen(1995) [31]	4832	1.4%
Padial(1996)[32]	566	6.5%
Cannan(1997) [33]	141	6%

Mueller (1998) [34]	333	8.1%
Chiang(1998) [35]	150	7.3%
Padial (1999)[36]	117	11.9%
Hernandz (1999) [24]	620	5.3%
Iung (2000) [25]	422	4%
Kang (2000) [37]	302	6.6%
Ben Farhat (2001) [38]	654	4.6%
Arora (2002) [39]	4850	1.4%
Konka (2003) [40]	1200	5.2%
Saadi (2005) [41]	356	6.1%
Jneid (2009) [42]	876	9.2%
Julio (2010) [43]	110	4.54%
Korkmaz (2011) [44]	311	1.6%

2- Mechanisms of injury :

The lesion mechanism of mitral regurgitation is determined by trans-thoracic ultrasound during percutaneous mitral dilatation. This may be confirmed by intraoperative analysis of the mitral valve.

Carpentier's classification of mitral insufficiency is based on analysis of the mechanism of leakage. Three types are distinguished (Figure 2):

- Type I: Valvular movements are normal.

The main lesion is dilatation of the annulus, which is often associated with deformation. Valvular perforations and tears are associated with this type.

- Type II: Valvular movements are exaggerated. The free edge of the valve leaflet protrudes beyond the plane of the annulus in systole.

The injuries in question are the breaking or stretching of ropes, and the breaking or stretching of pillars.

- Type III: Valvular movements are reduced by a lack of opening, or by excessive traction on the cords.

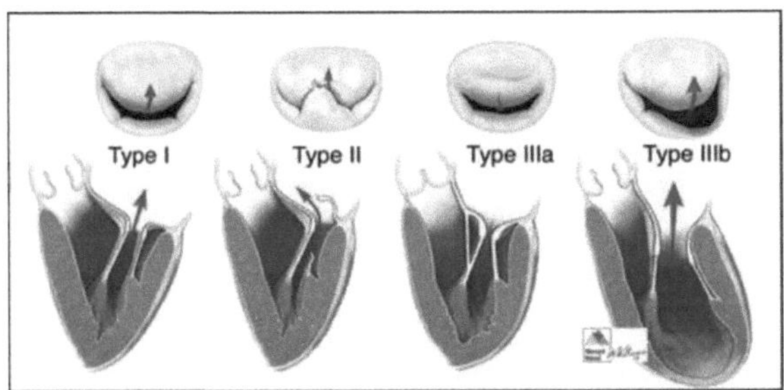

Figure 2: Carpentier functional classification of mitral insufficiency [45]. Traumatic mitral insufficiency after DMPC may be type I or type II, since it may be due to a tear in the anterior valvular leaflet or damage to the subvalvular apparatus [46].

In a pre-operative analysis of the mitral valve, C. Acar et al [47] identified four mechanisms of traumatic mitral leakage: rupture of a pillar, anterior leaflet tear, posterior leaflet tear and paracommissural tear.

Two other mechanisms have been described by other authors: cord rupture and excessive commissural opening [48].

- Tear of a valve leaflet: non-commissural tear (figure 3)

The majority of studies have found that valve tear is the predominant mechanism in the occurrence of severe mitral leakage after SCD [47,48, 49, 50, 51, 52, 53, 54]. They have also shown that severe mitral leakage occurs after the tearing of one or more valve segments, which are paradoxically the thinnest [55, 56].

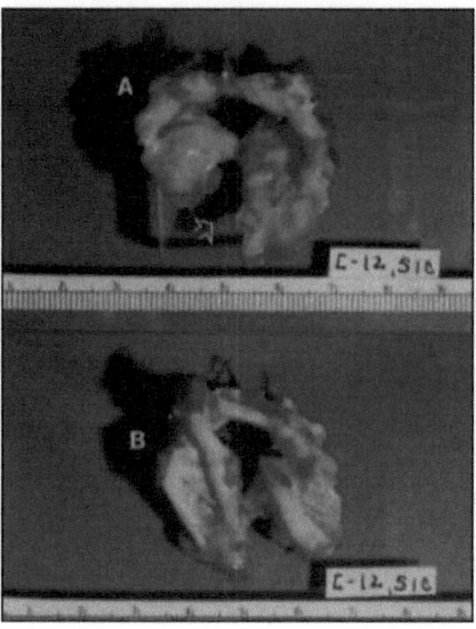

Figure 3: Surgical specimen of a tear in the greater mitral valve [57].

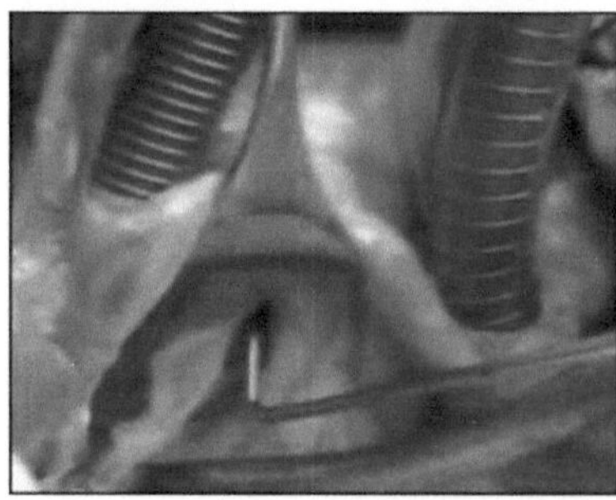

Figure 4: Tear in the GVM at segment A3.

In the series by Padial et al [32], 11 of the 13 patients operated on had a torn valve. Eleven patients had a Padial score greater than or equal to 3 for the torn valve, indicating a heterogeneous distribution of lesions, with the tear involving the thinnest segments of the valve.

Indeed, during inflation of the Inoue balloon, the pressure is exerted equally on the fused commissures and on the rest of the valve tissue. The result is less effective commissural release and a greater risk of valve tearing in the areas least resistant to the pressure exerted by the balloon.

The finest areas are the most vulnerable, especially :

- If they are adjacent to a very thick or calcified area that is resistant to pressure.

- If they are adjacent to a fused and/or calcified commissure.

- In the presence of 2 calcified commissures, both of which are resistant to pressure [58, 59, 60].

The thinner the vulnerable zone, the weaker it is. This has been highlighted in the Padial score. A valve segment is more likely to rupture if its thickness is between 4 and 5 mm (score 4) than if it is between 5 and 8 mm (score 3).

- **Anterior or posterior para-commissural tear:**

Paracommissural tears have been reported in the literature [30,61]. It is seen in cases of asymmetric remodelling of the two commissures. In this case, the thinner, less calcified commissure is ruptured. This tear may extend to the mitral annulus.

- **The breaking of a rope:**
Several authors [32, 33, 36, 38, 62, 63] have suggested that ruptured cords are the cause of severe MI, especially if the rupture is accompanied by valve prolapse.

There are two possible causes of rope failure:

- The tension exerted on a reworked sub-valvular apparatus during balloon dilation.

During DMPC using the Inoue balloon, after crossing the left ventricle, the distal balloon is withdrawn to anchor itself against the mitral valve. On withdrawal, it may deviate from the axis of the mitral-apex orifice of the left ventricle and become anchored in the cords. Inflation of the proximal balloon is accompanied by a slight rise in the distal balloon, which may rupture the cords [64, 65] (Figure 5).

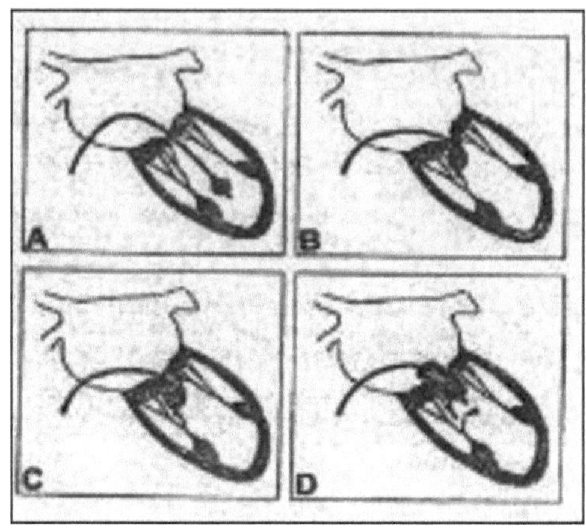

Figure 5: Mechanism responsible for rope failure [42].

- Pillar rupture (Figure 6)

This mechanism is rarely observed [32, 66, 67, 68].

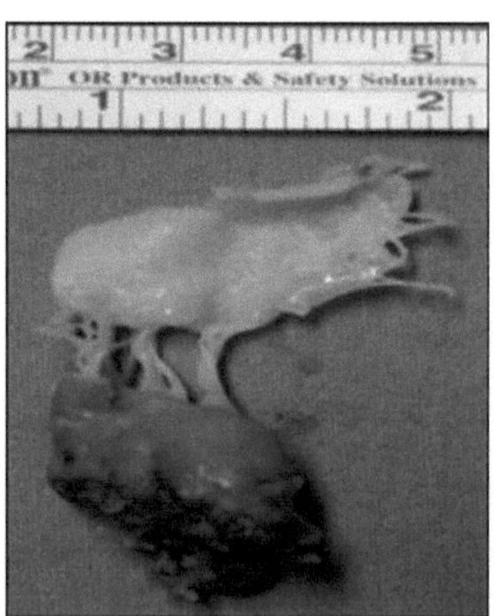

Figure 6: Surgical specimen of a traumatic abutment fracture [69].

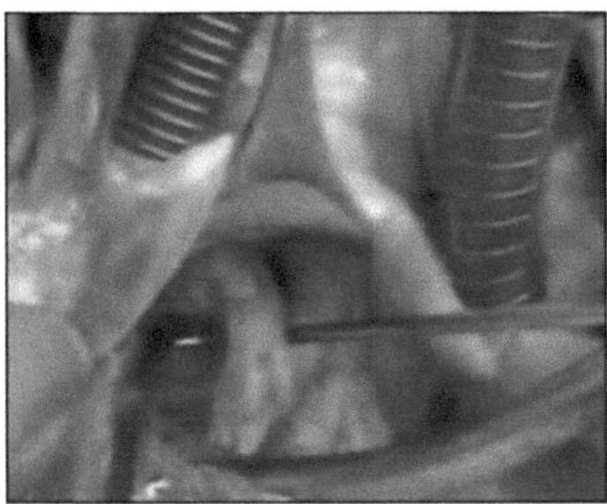

Figure 7: Total removal of the posterior abutment.

- Excessive opening of the commissures:

This mechanism is rarely described in the literature [63, 70, 71].

In the series by Vahanian [61] of 23 patients with traumatic MI, regurgitation was caused by a para-commissural tear of a valve leaflet in 20 cases, by rupture of a tendon cord in 2 cases, and by rupture of a papillary muscle in 1 case.

In the ICSC series [22], 2 significant mitral insufficiencies were due to a para-commissural tear close to the annulus, and one was due to a rupture of the cords.

In the series by Varma et al [72], 23 patients out of 1388 presented with acute MI. The mechanism in all cases was due to a valvular tear.

3- Contributing factors:

Prediction of the outcome of DMPC is multi-factorial, based on clinical, electrical and ultrasound criteria.

- **Functional impairment:** NYHA stages III and/or IV have been suggested to play a role in predicting MI [18, 72, 73].

- **Heart rate:** ACFA has been identified as a predictive factor for MI in several series [72, 73]. In other series [61, 74, 75, 76], there was no correlation.

Thus, the results of the literature are discordant with regard to the prediction of this parameter in the occurrence of a severe mitral leak.

- **Wilkins mitral morphology:** There is conflicting evidence in the literature regarding the validity of the Wilkins score in predicting the occurrence of traumatic MI.

In the series by Ben Farhat et al [38] of 654 patients, 4.6% had developed severe MI: the incidence of severe MI was 2.8% for a Wilkins score < 8, 8.6% for a score between 9 and 11, and 10.2% for a score > 12.

A Wilkins score > 8 was identified as a predictive factor for the occurrence of this complication (p=0.012).

In contrast, the majority of studies agree that the Wilkins ultrasound score taken as a whole does not predict the occurrence of mitral insufficiency [39, 76, 77, 78, 79, 80, 81, 82].

Mueller et al [34] compared a first group of 22 patients who developed a severe mitral leak with a second group of the same number who did not develop this complication. They found that the Wilkins score tended to be higher in the first group without reaching the significance threshold (7.68+/- 2.34 VS 6.91+/-1.93; p=0.24). This limitation may be due to the lack of study of commissural morphology using this score.

Padial et al [32] have shown that a Wilkins score greater than 10 is a powerful predictive factor for the occurrence of severe MI, with a sensitivity of 83% and a specificity of 100%.

Konka et al [40] found that the willkins score did not predict the complication, as there was no significant difference between the severe MI group and the group without severe MI (8.23+/-1.9vs 7.49+/-1.5; p=0.22).

- **Valvular mobility:** Valvular mobility may be influenced by calcifications, commissural fusion or damage to the subvalvular apparatus [82]. As a result, it has rarely been used by authors to predict the occurrence of a mitral leak after DMPC.

Karasuski et al [83] compared a 1st group of 268 young patients with a second group of 55 patients aged over 65 years and found no significant difference in the occurrence of severe MI post DMPC despite the 2nd group having less mobile valves (p =0.005).

Similarly, Mueller et al [43], comparing a group of 22 patients who had developed a severe mitral leak with a second group of the same number who had not developed a leak, found no difference in valve mobility (p=0.3).

- **Valvular thickening:** There are few series in the literature which have studied the exclusive role of this parameter.

Mueller et al [43] found no relationship between valve thickening and the occurrence of severe mitral leakage. In addition, Krasuski et al [84] found that patients aged over 65 had significantly thicker valves than younger patients (p=0.001), while the rate of post-procedural severe MI was not statistically higher.

- **Valvular calcifications:** There is conflicting evidence in the literature.

In the series by Krasuski et al [84], valve calcification was not associated with the occurrence of severe MI. Indeed, the authors found that patients aged over 65 had more calcified valves than younger patients and that this difference was clearly significant (p<0.0001). However, they did not find a statistically significant difference in the rate of severe post-procedural MI between the 2 age groups.

Hung et al [85], and Vahanian et al [29], found that valvular calcifications were one of the predictive factors for severe MI. These same results were found by Iung et al [86, 87].

- **Changes in the mitral subvalvular apparatus:** The role of changes in the ASV in predicting mitral leakage after SCD has not been well studied and remains a controversial subject. Several ultrasound scores have been established to assess the ASV; the best known and most widely used is the Wilkins score.

Lau et al [88] and Chen et al [89] have shown a correlation between damage to the ASV and the occurrence of mitral leakage.

Similarly, Konka et al [49] concluded that ASV changes were predictive of severe MI. In their series of 1200 patients who had undergone DMPC, 62 (5.2%) were complicated by a leak > grade 3. These patients were compared with a group of the same number with procedural success. The ASV was significantly more severely affected in the first group.

In the series of 566 patients by Padial et al [32], VSA was assessed according to the Wilkins criteria. The score was significantly higher in patients who had developed this complication.

Chen et al [89] reported a relationship between the severity of ASV damage and the mitral surface area obtained after DMPC, but found that ASV was not a predictive factor for the occurrence of severe mitral leakage. According to these authors, the presence of thickened and fused cords may predispose to their rupture without creating a severe MI.

Thus, the results of the literature concerning the predictive value of VSA are discordant. This wide variability in results has been linked to the non-quantitative and therefore subjective nature of the Wilkins score assessment of VSA.

- Mitral morphology according to Padial: The Padial score is an ultrasound score established by Padial [32, 36] to predict the occurrence of severe MI after DMPC according to the anatomical state of the mitral apparatus. This score is based on the heterogeneity of the distribution of valve thickening and calcifications rather than their severity, on the symmetry or asymmetry of commissural lesions, and on the severity of ASV remodelling.

It was first proposed in 1996 to predict severe MI after double-balloon DMPC [32]. The values of this score vary between 4 and 16.

In 1999, Padial et al [32] applied this score in a series of 117 patients who had undergone DMPC with the Inoue balloon. 14 patients developed MI > grade 3. Fourteen patients developed MI > grade 3. The Padial score was higher in the MI group than in the no MI group. In addition, large valve, small valve, commissure and ASV scores were also higher in patients with severe MI. The threshold value for prediction was 10 and the sensitivity of this score for predicting severe MI was 82%, specificity 91%; while the Wilkins score was not significantly different between the 2 groups.

This score has therefore proved superior to the Wilkins score in predicting outcomes by studying commissural morphology.

Since the main mechanism of action of DMPC is the separation of fused commissures, the presence of significant fibrosis or commissural calcifications will be a predictive factor for failure of the procedure due to aggravation of the MI [46, 90, 91].

Various series of open-heart commissurotomy surgeries, such as that of Gross et al [92], and studies of patients operated for mitral insufficiency after DMPC [93], such as that of Miche et al [98], have shown that the mitral valves were heterogeneously thickened, that one or both commissures were calcified, and that the ASV was thickened, fused and shortened.

Similarly, Reifart et al [94] dilated in vitro 15 valves excised from patients who had undergone valve replacement for rheumatic MR. In 20% of cases, they noted the occurrence of a valvular tear involving the least affected segments of the mitral valves, the thickness of which was very heterogeneous and one or both commissures of which were fibrous and calcified. They concluded that severe MI after DMPC depends above all on the heterogeneity of the distribution of lesions rather than their severity.

- **Pulmonary arterial hypertension:** Pulmonary arterial hypertension (PAH) is also a factor correlated with poor results from DMPC [95]. In fact, the greater the degree of PAH, the greater the technical difficulty due to dilatation of the right atrium, which complicates the trans septal puncture stage, and an often tighter mitral surface, which increases the risk of mitral insufficiency [96].

Indeed, Pande et al [97] in a series of 46 patients with severe MI post DMPC, found that only 11 patients required urgent surgery within less than 6 hours. Comparing these patients with the others, they concluded that pre-procedural PAH greater than 76 mm Hg or post-procedural PAH greater than 77 mm Hg were predictive factors of severe surgical MI with a sensitivity and specificity of 72% and 63%, and 100% and 90%, respectively.

- **Advanced age:** Older patients often have more unfavourable anatomical forms due to the longer evolution and repeated attacks of AAR with highly calcified forms and significant remodelling of the sub-valvular apparatus [15, 98]. These patients have significant co-morbidities, which limits the risks involved in choosing the balloon and inflation pressure.

- **Pre-procedural mitral surface area:** Several authors have studied the relationship between SM prior to DMPC and the occurrence of severe post-procedural mitral leak. The data in the literature are very discordant.

Palacios et al [99] carried out a multi-variate study in a series of 939 DMPC in search of factors predictive of severe mitral leakage and showed that SM before DMPC was highly predictive.

Hernandez et al [24], in a series of 561 patients who had undergone DMPC, showed that the mitral surface area before the procedure is a predictive factor for post-procedural severe mitral leakage. Indeed, when the pre-procedural MS is between 0.8 and 1 cm^2 , the risk of the complication occurring is multiplied by 2; and when it is < 0.79 cm2 , the risk is multiplied by 4.5. A mitral surface area greater than 1 cm^2 is correlated with good results [100].

lung et al [106] in a series of 422 patients, showed that pre-procedural SM was an independent predictor of severe MI (p=0.0005).

However, in a study of 600 patients by Arora et al [17], pre-procedural SM was not found to be predictive of severe mitral leakage.

Thus, the results of the literature are discordant with regard to the prediction of this parameter in the occurrence of a severe mitral leak.

- The grade of mitral insufficiency prior to DMPC: The data in the literature are also discordant. Padial et al [36] showed that the degree of pre-existing MI was not predictive of severe mitral leakage.

Alfonso et al [30] compared a first group of 102 patients with minimal pre-procedural MI with a second group of 186 patients without initial MI. Minimal pre-procedural MI was not predictive of severe mitral leak after DMPC.

Furthermore, in the series by Ben Farhat et al [26], involving 463 patients, pre-procedural MI was identified as a predictive factor for the complication (p=0.006).

In the series by Jneid et al [42], the degree of pre-procedural MI was an independent factor in the development of large MI. Thus, 22% of patients with moderate pre-procedural MI developed a large MI compared with 13% of patients with mild MI and 5% of patients with no MI.

- The mean gradient between the OG and the LV and the size of the OG: Iung et al [25], in a series of 232 patients, did not find these parameters to be predictive of severe MI.

On the other hand, Mailer et al [102] have shown that the size of the OG and the mean OG-VG gradient are predictive factors for the development of post-DMPC MI.

- Left ventricular function: Sancho et al [103] showed that left ventricular dysfunction was a predictive factor for the occurrence of severe mitral leak. On the other hand, Sutaria et al [52], in a series of 300 DMPC, found no relationship between left ventricular function and the occurrence of a mitral leak.

- DMPC redux: DMPC redux is still indicated for elderly patients with multiple co-morbidities and a high operative risk. In the literature, few studies have been devoted to iterative mitral dilatation because of the small number of patients and the fact that the decision is often taken surgically. The results of mitral redux dilatation depend largely on the mechanism of restenosis. The most favourable forms are those with bi-commissural refusion, whereas the most unfavourable forms are those with a highly remodelled sub-valvular apparatus with sub-valvular narrowing.

In the majority of published studies of percutaneous mitral re-dilation, remodelling of the valvular and subvalvular apparatus was greater than in de novo dilation [25, 27]. This remodelling, together with the presence of commissural calcifications, has also been reported to be predictive of mitral leakage [104].

In a series on percutaneous mitral re-dilation, Lung B et al [25] observed that a MI was created or aggravated in 44% of cases with a severe mitral leak in 4% of cases.

Hernandez et al [24] observed a worsening or creation of a mitral leak in 23% of their patients.

    - **The DMPC technique used:** According to Ben Farhat et al [26], the Inoue technique has been identified as being associated with a higher risk of severe mitral insufficiency: 10.5% compared with 5% with the double balloon technique.

For Nobuyoshi [105], the incidence of MI is higher in series of valvuloplasty with double balloons than in those with Inoue balloons. For other authors, the two techniques have comparable results [46, 106, 107, 108, 109].

    - **The diameter of the balloon used and the number of inflations**: According to Herman [110], there is no significant correlation between the size of the balloon used and the degree of mitral insufficiency.

Inoue [111] also believes that there is no real correlation between balloon size and the degree of mitral insufficiency, but suggests that severe MI may be related to the use of balloons that are too large. On the other hand, Zaibag [112], Padial [36] and Sung Hung [113] have shown that there is an increased risk of MI with increasing balloon size. The amount of inflation is also a factor in the occurrence of severe MI [114,115].

    - **Biological markers of inflammation: C-reactive protein/sedimentation rate/leukocyte count:** Increased C-reactive protein levels in patients with chronic rheumatic disease have been reported, and are described as evidence of an inflammatory process [116]. Elevated levels are correlated with procedural failure.

An elevated sedimentation rate and leukocyte count at the time of DMPC is also correlated with a high rate of MI [117].

V- Diagnosis of acute mitral insufficiency :

Intra-procedural ultrasound makes an important contribution to the detection of mitral regurgitation.

1- Clinical manifestations :

The clinical tolerance of mitral insufficiency varies from one patient to another, which explains the need or not to refer the patient to the surgeon and the degree of urgency of the surgical procedure [118].

This is a picture of acute pulmonary oedema of varying severity, depending on the degree of pre-existing dilatation of the OG and the size of the leak caused by the trauma to the mitral valve, with the appearance of dyspnoea and a peak holo-systolic murmur. A state of shock with a fall in blood pressure and tachycardia may also be seen.

2- Special case of HMPD in pregnant women:

The association of heart disease and pregnancy is not exceptional. Its prevalence varies between 0.1 and 4% [119].

Physiological changes in haemodynamics during pregnancy are the main cause of decompensation of mitral stenosis.

In the case of tight MR in pregnant women, the increase in blood volume, tachycardia and impediment to ventricular filling lead to pulmonary arterial hypertension and worsening of dyspnoea, or even PAO and cardiogenic shock [120]. This condition leads to maternal-foetal hypoxia with repercussions on foetal development.

Percutaneous dilatation is the treatment of choice for tight mitral stenosis in pregnant women. It can be performed from the twelfth week of pregnancy to minimise the risk of teratogenesis, while taking the necessary precautions by protecting the patient's abdomen with a lead waistcoat extended from the mother's diaphragm to the pelvis.

The results are favourable for the mother, with a reduction in foetal morbidity and mortality. However, the series published on DMPC in pregnant women have focused on a limited number of cases.

The low incidence of severe MI in pregnant women explains the statistical difficulty in identifying predictive factors for its occurrence. The hypothesis that osteogenic impregnation of valve tissue during pregnancy exposes pregnant women to a higher risk of valve tears after dilatation is not borne out by a review of the literature, since the frequency of severe MI is equivalent to, if not lower than, that in the non-pregnant context.

In series published in the literature, the incidence of severe MI is low [121, 122, 123, 124]. In the series by Gamra et al [121], the incidence was 1.6%. In the series by Ben Farhat et al [122] only one patient had DMPC complicated by severe MI (2.3%).

- Contribution of trans-thoracic echocardiography :

It allows a positive diagnosis of mitral leakage to be made using Doppler by finding the jet of very high velocity holo-systolic regurgitation in the OG, or even in the pulmonary veins.

TTE can also be used to identify the lesions caused by the dilatation procedure, thus defining the mechanism of the leak and classifying it according to Carpentier's classification. The severity of the MI can be assessed by :

- Quantitative assessment using the PISA method, which is the reference method for measuring the surface area of the regurgitant orifice and the volume regurgitated at each systole.

A grade 3 MI is defined by a regurgitant volume between 45 and 60 ml, and a grade 4 MI is defined by a regurgitant volume > 60 ml.

-        Semi-quantitative evaluation by assessing the extent of the leak in the OG, the width of the jet at the origin and the change in flow in the pulmonary veins as a result of MI.

-        Detection of any significant PAH, and exploration of the tricuspid valve.

- Contribution of transesophageal echocardiography :

Pre-operative TEE provides a better means of studying the mechanism responsible for mitral leakage, since it is more sensitive and specific than TEE.

Intraoperative TEE is vital for elucidating the mechanism of regurgitation and planning the management strategy.

Intra-operative assessment of MI is modified by anaesthesia, which tends to reduce its importance by lowering blood pressure and filling. For example, MI falls by 1 to 2 degrees in half of patients simply because they are asleep [125].

Figure 8 [126] shows an ultrasound image of a GVM tear on TEE. Three-dimensional TEE allows the exact location of the valve lesion to be determined.

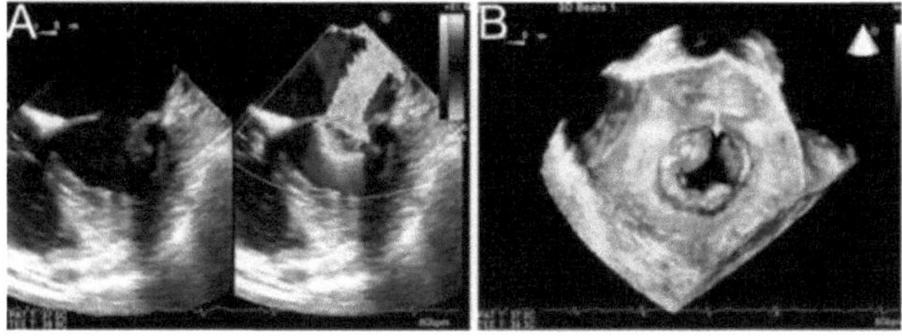

Figure 8: Ultrasound image of a large mitral leak due to a GVM tear [126].

(A) Severe MI associated with a GVM tear.

(B) TEE in three-dimensional mode showing the exact location of the tear (A2).

VI- Treatment of acute mitral insufficiency :

1- Medical treatment :

- 2014 American Heart Association / American College of Cardiology recommendations [127]:

Systemic vasodilators can be used to reduce regurgitant volume. Placement of an intra-aortic counterpulsation balloon is useful in the treatment of acute mitral insufficiency. It reduces left ventricular afterload and lowers aortic diastolic and mean pressure. It therefore makes it possible to stabilise haemodynamic constants while awaiting surgical repair.

- Recommendations of the European Society of Cardiology 2012 [128]:

Diuretics and nitrates help to reduce filling pressures.

Sodium nitroprusside reduces afterload and the regurgitation fraction.

Positive inotropic agents and the counterpulsation balloon are indicated in cases of arterial hypotension. The aim is to increase pressure in the aortic root and maintain it above pulmonary arterial pressure to improve perfusion of the coronary arteries.

2- Surgical treatment :

The operation is performed under extracorporeal circulation (ECG). It may be a conservative procedure or a valve replacement, depending on the extent of rheumatic or traumatic valve lesions.

- Recommendations of the European Society of Cardiology 2012 [128]:

Surgery is indicated as an emergency measure in patients with severe acute mitral leaks, after stabilisation of the haemodynamic state using an intra-aortic counterpulsation balloon, positive inotropes and vasodilators.

- 2014 American Heart Association / American College of Cardiology recommendations [127]:

Surgery for acute mitral insufficiency is indicated as an emergency procedure when regurgitation is severe in a symptomatic patient. The degree of urgency depends on the patient's haemodynamic tolerance.

Surgical treatment is therefore indicated for massive leaks (grade III to IV). In some cases, the operation is not urgent, and is planned in the weeks following the procedure. In most cases, however, clinical intolerance means that emergency surgery is required.

- Pre-operative assessment and particularities of pre-operative anaesthesia [129] :

In the case of major leaks caused by traumatic damage to the mitral valve, total blood volume is increased in order to maintain an effective systemic flow rate, given the loss of volume in the back-and-forth flow between the LV and the OG. Hypovolaemia reduces systemic flow proportionately more than the regurgitated fraction. Tolerance to hypovolaemia is low and preload must be maintained at normal to high levels.

As the LV functions as a cavity with two outlets, the volume regurgitated is a direct function of the resistance to ejection. Systemic arterial resistance must be kept low. Arterial vasodilatation is therefore necessary, hence the use of vasodilating agents such as isoflurane, nitroprusside and phenotolamine.

Contractility must be kept high to ensure systolic flow. It is improved by inotropic agents without alpha effects such as dobutamine, isoprenaline, amrinone, and milrinone. Milrinone is preferred to dobutamine, norepinephrine and levosimendan [130]. In the event of difficulty, intra-aortic counterpulsation is very effective in relieving LV pressure, reducing MI and improving coronary perfusion.

In addition, vasopressin may be required in cases of shock with vasodilatation and pulmonary arterial hypertension.

Positive pressure mechanical ventilation improves left-sided flow as long as venous return to the right heart remains assured. Emptying from the lungs into the OG is accelerated, anterograde mitral flow is increased and transmural pressure in the atrium is reduced [131].

The Swan Ganz pulmonary catheter is very useful for this surgery in order to regulate fluid administration, monitor the evolution of pressures in the OG and be able to assess the anterograde systolic volume. After bypass, it is useful for managing LV haemodynamic support, since correction of the mitral leak imposes difficult conditions on the LV: increased afterload and reduced preload [132].

Reduction of right ventricular afterload using pulmonary vasodilators is also recommended after surgery.

- Thoracic approach :

Vertical median sternotomy: The skin incision extends from the sternal fork to the xiphoid process (figure 9), then the sternum is incised with a saw.

This route allows rapid and easy installation of the bypass graft and easy access to the mitral valve [133].

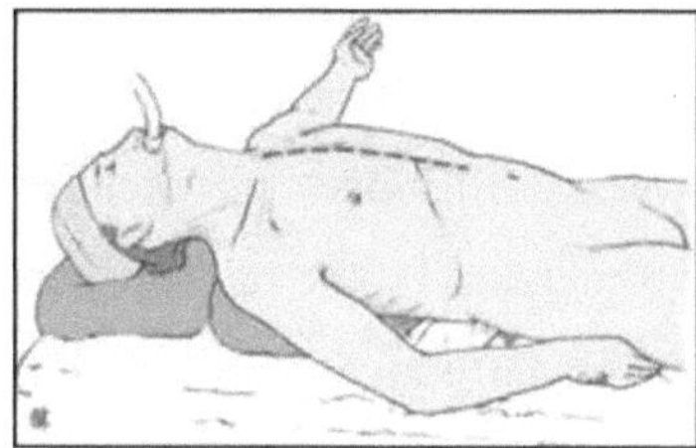

Figure 9. Vertical median sternotomy [133].

Right anterolateral thoracotomy: This approach has aesthetic advantages, especially in women.

The skin incision is located in the submammary fold. It measures approximately 6 cm and will be hidden by the breast. The thorax is opened in the fourth intercostal space (figure 10).

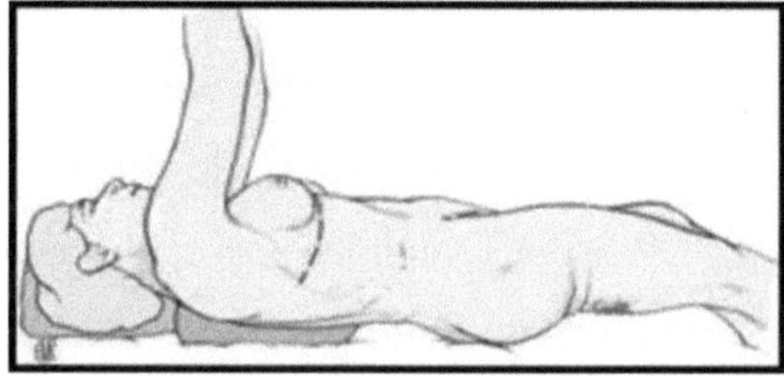

Figure 10: Right anterolateral thoracotomy [133].

Mini-sternotomy: The advantage of this approach is that it reduces post-operative pain and the risk of infection, as well as the average length of hospital stay, and to a lesser extent offers an aesthetic advantage, without compromising the surgical result.

The opening of the sternum is in the shape of an inverted "L". It begins below Louis' angle and extends as far as the xiphoid process. Some teams add a second incision opposite the second right intercostal space, giving a "T-shaped" incision (Figure 11).

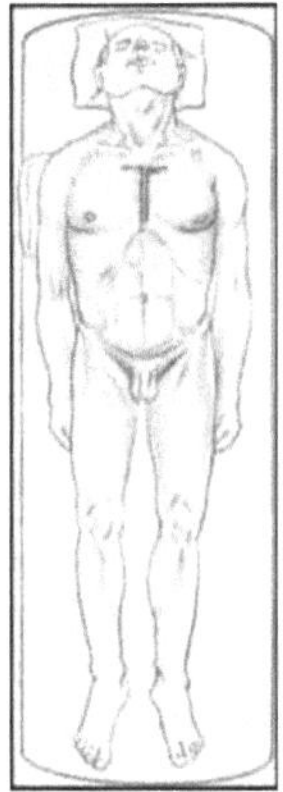

Figure 11: Inverted L or T mini-sternotomy [133].

Video surgery: Video-assisted mitral surgery is a new minimally invasive approach that reduces post-operative pain, cuts down on bleeding and blood transfusions, reduces the duration of mechanical ventilation and the length of hospital stay, with a lower risk of complications.

and aesthetic benefits. It may or may not be combined with an anterolateral thoracotomy.

The limitations are high cost and technical difficulty.

- **Extracorporeal circulation :**

Extracorporeal circulation is installed between the two vena cava and the ascending aorta. The two vena cava must be cannulated in order to squeeze the cava lakes and dry out the right cavities, and consequently the return via the pulmonary veins.

It is essential to obtain an empty left atrium. A dual current needle is placed in the ascending aorta to administer cardioplegia and purges. Inotropic support is almost always required for emergence from bypass. This should be provided by non-alpha amines: dobutamine, milrinone. The addition of an arterial vasodilator may occasionally be necessary when systemic arterial resistance is too high [134].

The presence of pulmonary hypertension creates a risk of right ventricular decompensation at the end of bypass surgery.

- **Approach to the mitral valve :**

The route of exposure of the mitral valve depends on whether or not there is dilatation of the left atrium.

Left auriculotomy in Sondergaardt's sulcus: This is the route most frequently used when the left atrium is dilated. The opening is made 2 to 3 mm behind Sondergaardt's sulcus (Figure 12).

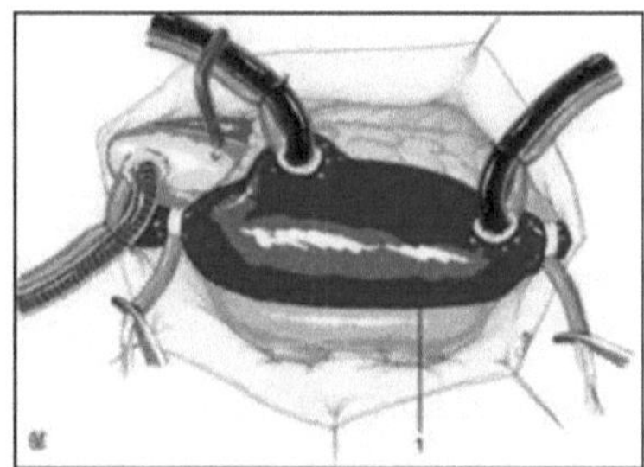

Figure 12: Left auriculotomy in the Sondergaardt sulcus [133].

The trans-septal bi-atrial approach: This involves opening the right superior pulmonary vein and ascending through an oblique incision in the right atrium. The interatrial septum is then incised in a curve, avoiding the area of Hiss' bundle (Figure 13).

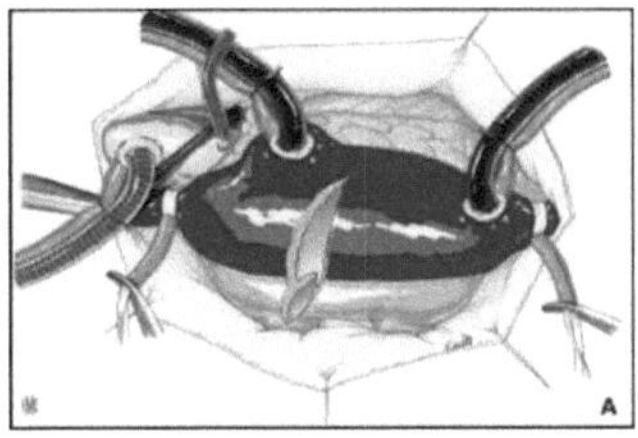

Figure 13: Incision of the right superior pulmonary vein [133].

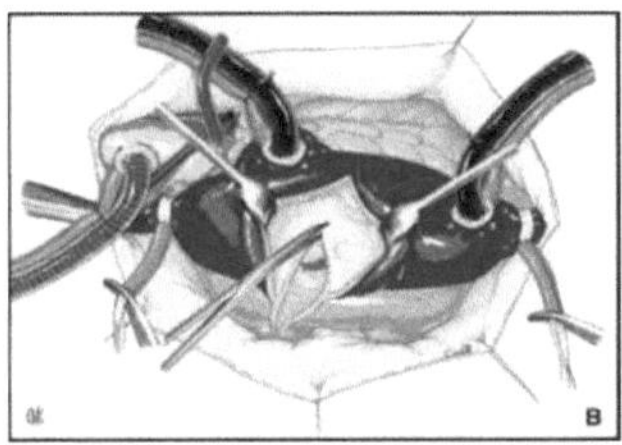

Figure 14: Incision of the atrial septum [133].

The vertical trans-septal approach: This involves making an incision in the right atrium parallel to the atrioventricular groove, or obliquely, and then opening the left atrium via a vertical septal incision (Figure 15).

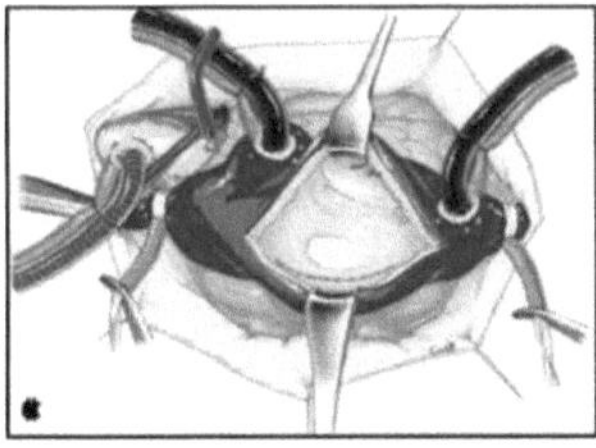

Figure 15: Trans-septal bi-atrial approach [133].

- Comparison of ultrasound data and intraoperative findings :

Macroscopic examination of the valve leaflets, commissures, annulus and sub-valvular apparatus enables rheumatic and traumatic lesions to be identified and compared with the preoperative ultrasound data (Figure 16).

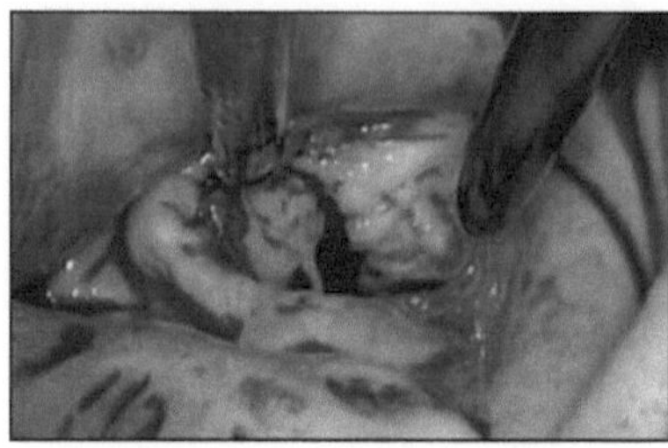

Figure 16: Intraoperative image of an A2 tear [126].

This discrepancy may be explained by the fact that TTE is not very sensitive and may underestimate the severity of lesions and the extent of mitral leakage [53]. Compared with conventional trans-thoracic ultrasound, trans-oesophageal ultrasound has the advantage of bypassing the thoracic cavity and the lungs, which allows the heart to be approached directly behind the OG and high image definition to be obtained. For this reason, it is more sensitive in terms of the precise study of anatomical lesions and the extent of regurgitation (Figure 17).

Figure 17: Ultrasound and operative findings in mitral valve lesions following DMPC [135].

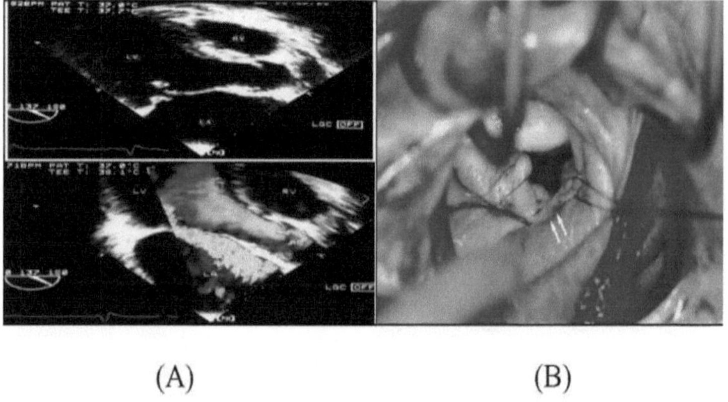

(A)   (B)

(A) Multi-plane OCT showing a large MI reaching the roof of the OG and a tear in the PVM.

(B) Concordance of operative and ultrasound data: the arrow shows the exact location of the PVM tear (P2).

- Valve procedures :

Mitral valve replacement: The choice of the type of prosthesis to be implanted depends on the patient's age, heart rhythm and the presence or absence of contraindications to anticoagulant treatment.

Mechanical prostheses have the advantage of durability and good haemodynamic performance. However, they carry the risk of thromboembolic and haemorrhagic complications, as well as infective endocarditis. Bioprostheses have the advantage of not requiring lifelong anti-coagulant treatment, but their major disadvantage is the high risk of degeneration.

The valve replacement technique: The valve may be totally or partially resected, leaving the posterior leaflet intact (Figure 18).

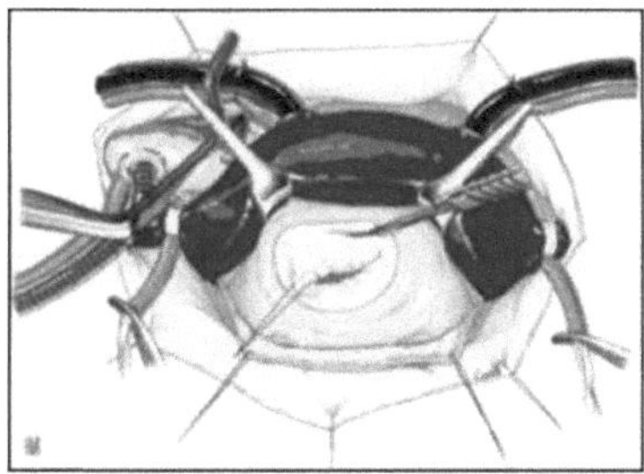

Figure 18: Resection of the valve by detachment of its annular insertion [133].

Preservation of the sub-valvular apparatus improves post-operative haemodynamic results.

To choose the size of the prosthesis, a tester must be placed completely in the mitral orifice. It must pass freely through the orifice (Figure 19). If the prosthesis is too large, there is a risk of rupture of the annulus and compression of the circumflex artery.

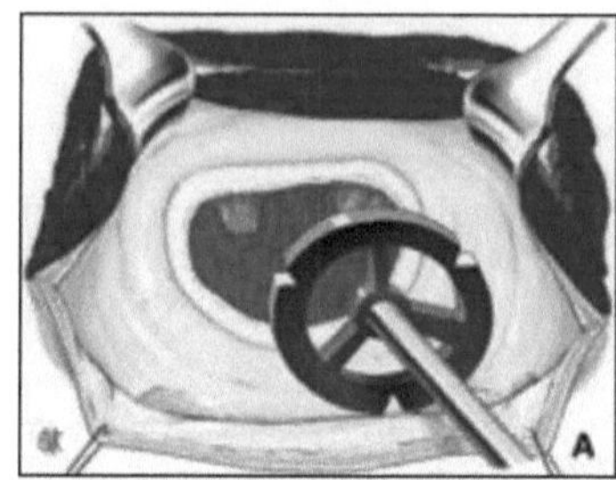

Figure 19: Choice of prosthesis size by a tester [133].

In the case of mechanical prostheses, the wings may be in an anatomical or anti-anatomical position. For biological prostheses, they have three equidistant biological tissue fixation posts, whether pericardial or porcine.

The prosthesis can be attached using separate, simple, U-shaped or X-shaped stitches, or by overlocking. U-shaped stitches supported on felt splints (pledjet) are used when the ring is fragile, and particularly in the event of traumatic rupture of the ring during the procedure.

Conservative surgery of the mitral valve: Despite advances in mitral surgery and improvements in surgical techniques allowing greater conservation of the subvalvular apparatus, mitral valvuloplasty remains the only technique that truly respects the subvalvular apparatus [86].

However, the indications for mitral plasty are limited in cases of traumatic MI due to rheumatic valve disease because of the changes and calcifications of the leaflets and cords, and the difficulty of repairing additional traumatic lesions [72].

The aim of mitral reconstructive surgery is to restore normal function to the valve. This can be achieved using a range of techniques adapted to the valve dysfunction and lesions.

Functional analysis is the first important step in reconstructive surgery. Its aim is to analyse the valve dysfunction, locate it segment by segment and identify the lesion responsible for the dysfunction.

This functional analysis can be carried out pre-operatively by ultrasound, or during the operation. Several dysfunctions may coexist in the same mitral valve, since it combines rheumatic and traumatic lesions.

This segmental analysis makes it possible to classify the MI, predict its feasibility for plasty, and plan the techniques to be used.

Placement of a Carpentier annulus in the case of traumatic post-DMPC MI is not systematic, but rather depends on the type of lesion. It is used not only for anti-reflux purposes, but above all to reinforce the valve sutures, particularly in the case of PVM tears or paracommissural tears [135].

There are two types of prosthetic rings:

- Semi-rigid rings: open in the middle of their anterior portion

- Flexible rings: a more recent development, these are either flexible in all their portions, or they have a flexible portion at the posterior and commissural level and a rigid anterior portion.

Two measurements are used to select the ring size:

- The inter-commissural distance: this is measured between the two points placed at each commissure.

- The height of the anterior sheet: this is measured by pulling the entire anterior sheet through the main ropes with a hook. This height must be completely covered by the measurer.

The ring is fitted using U-shaped stitches of 2/0 braided wire.

In the series by Acar [54], 10 patients underwent mitral plasty and 6 mitral valve replacement. For patients who underwent reconstructive surgery, repair of traumatic lesions was combined with the insertion of a prosthetic ring to reinforce the valve sutures in 8 cases.

This suture technique with ring reinforcement was also used in the Abid series [136].

Prolapse of the posterior leaflet may be secondary to traumatic rupture of a cord or abutment during the procedure.

In this case, the repair consists of a quadrangular resection of the prolapsed area, folding of the annulus and suturing of the valve margins using separate stitches (Figure 20). A prosthetic ring is then inserted.

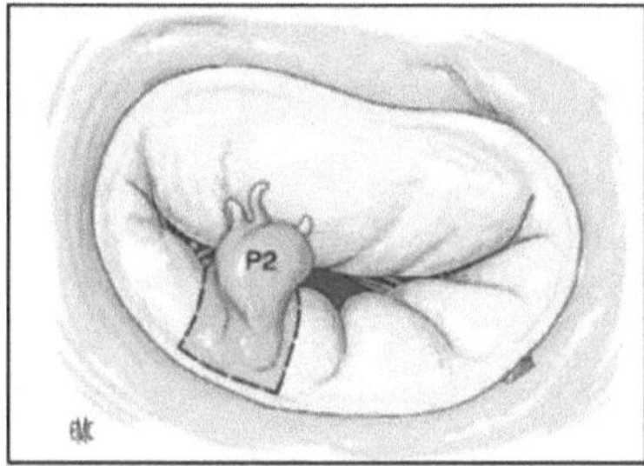

Figure 20: Quadrangular resection for prolapse of a posterior leaflet [136].

The technique used depends on the lesions responsible for the prolapse of the anterior leaflet. In the case of ruptured cords, the conservative surgical techniques are :

- Triangular resection: As this technique did not produce good results, it was abandoned in favour of two other techniques (Figure 21).

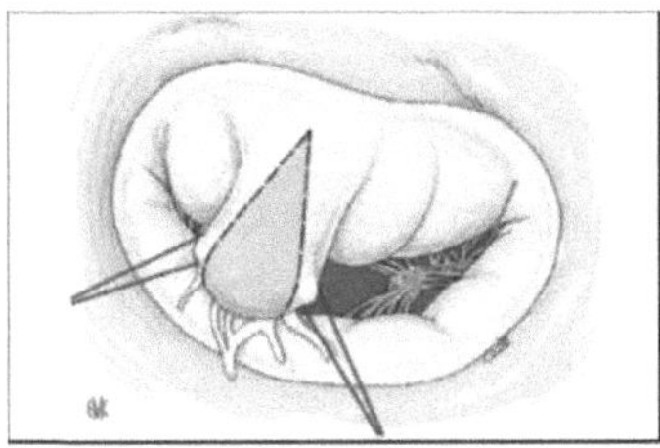

Figure 21: Triangular resection of a prolapsed segment of the anterior valve [136].

- Transposition of cords: This involves transferring a solid cord from the posterior leaflet opposite the anterior prolapse to the free edge of the anterior leaflet.

This cord is detached from the posterior leaflet by excising a piece of valve tissue and then sutured firmly to the free edge of the anterior leaflet at the level of the cord break (Figure 22).

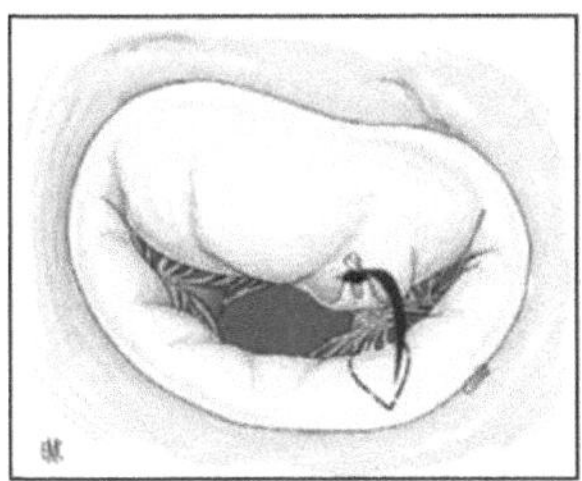

Figure 22: Transposition of the cord from the posterior leaflet to the free edge of the anterior leaflet [136].

- Marginalisation of secondary cords: If there is a solid secondary cord close to the prolapse, it can be attached to the free edge using two or three trans-fixing stitches.

- Placement of artificial cords: These are made of GORTEX. They can be inserted into the anterior or posterior leaflet (figure 23).

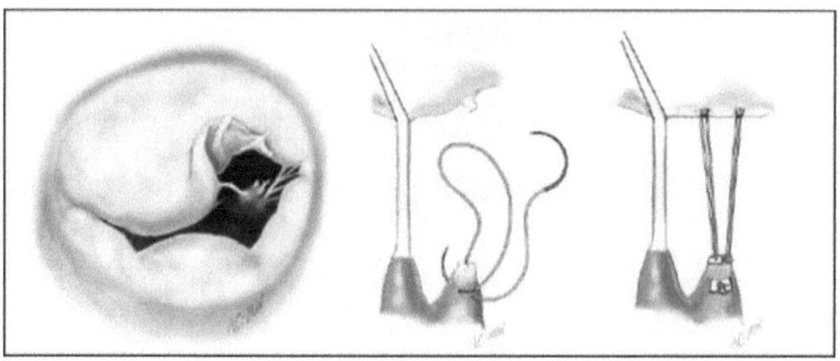

Figure 23: Installation of GORTEX ropes [136].

- In the event of abutment rupture: Reimplantation of a ruptured abutment can be carried out directly at the level of the remaining abutment or at the level of the left ventricular wall.

- In the case of commissural prolapse: The most frequent mechanism is cord rupture (in 45% of cases) and it mainly involves the posterior commissure (75%) and less often the anterior commissure (25%). Surgical treatment is conservative in the majority of cases.

The simplest and most common technique (50% of cases) is closure of the commissure (Figure 24), in the absence of secondary mitral stenosis. It is also possible to use artificial cords in this indication, to resect the anterior or posterior valve leaflet adjacent to the commissure, or even to replace the entire commissure with a partial homograft (Figure 25).

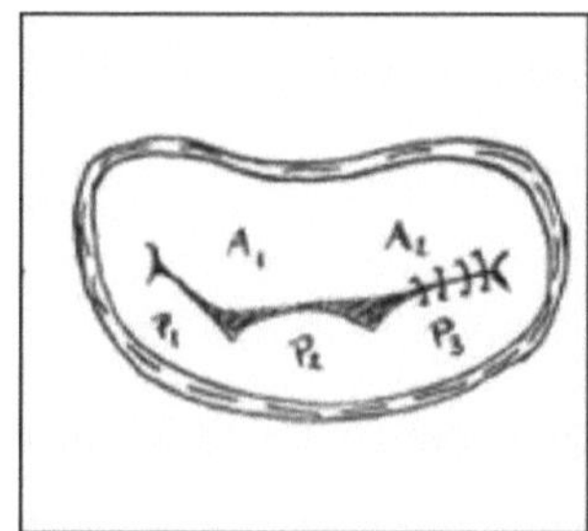

Figure 24: Simple closure of the commissure.

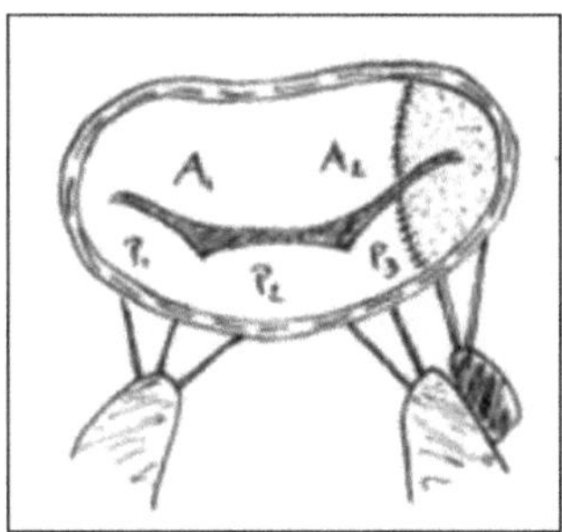

Figure 25: Partial homograft in the posterior commissural position.

In the series by Vahanian [18], 5 patients underwent surgery for acute massive MI post DMPC. Four patients underwent commissuroplasty and one patient underwent RVM.

- Reconstruction in the case of a torn valve leaflet: Two techniques are of interest in this context:

- Use of an autologous pericardium patch: the patch replaces a loss of valve substance and retains a certain amount of valve tissue (figure 26).

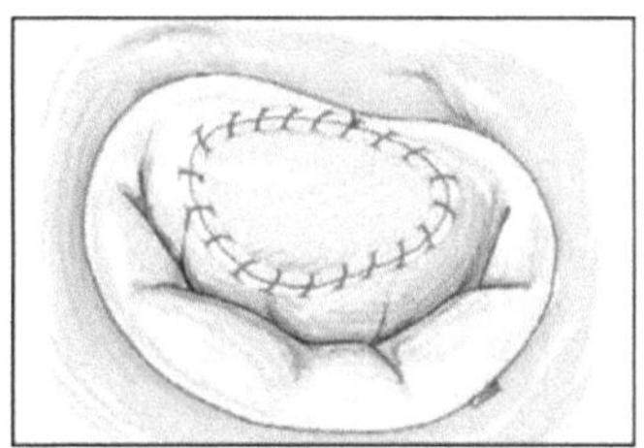

Figure 26: Reconstruction of a tear in a valve leaflet using a pericardial patch [136].

Acar [53] reported in his series 2 cases of anterior leaflet tear in which he performed a wide commissurotomy, fenestration of the fused cords, longitudinal cleavage of the leaflets and repair of the anterior leaflet tear with a patch of autologous pericardium treated for 15 minutes with Glutaraldehyde.

In the series by Abid [136], 1 patient with a traumatic tear of the large mitral valve underwent repair with an untreated autologous pericardial patch that progressed to restenosis.

Treatment of the pericardium with glutaraldehyde therefore appears necessary to prevent retraction of the pericardium and progression to mitral restenosis.

- Direct suture: This technique is mainly used for para-commissural tears. This technique has also been reported by Acar [53] in 1 case of a medial tear of the posterior leaflet: this was treated by minimal resection of the prolapsed area followed by direct suture of the valve. A double commissurotomy was also performed and a Carpentier ring was inserted to reinforce the valve sutures. This technique was also used in Abid's series [136].

- Reconstruction in cases of para-commissural tears: In the series by Acar [53], 7 cases of para-commissural tears were described. These patients had valves with little remodelling and underwent mitral commissurotomy. The pillars were cleaved. The para-commissural tear was repaired by direct suture. In 5 cases, a Carpentier ring was inserted.

- Percutaneous repair of mitral insufficiency: These new techniques are currently being studied. The majority of these techniques are based on well-established surgical procedures, which have progressed towards a less invasive approach. However, the anatomical complexity of the mitral valve and the diversity of pathological conditions make it difficult to develop these techniques. At present, these treatments should only be offered to patients considered to be at high risk of surgery or inoperable. As a result, these techniques have no place in the treatment of severe MI post DMPC.

- Mitral valve plasty or replacement: In acute traumatic post-CPMS MI, mitral damage often occurs in rheumatic and remodelled valves, and traumatic lesions are often extensive. This condition appears to be less amenable to valve repair than other MI aetiologies due to major calcifications, reduced leaflet mobility and extensive remodelling of the valvular or subvalvular tissue [136, 137, 138], and often requires valve replacement [80, 81, 82]. In addition, repair should not be performed in patients with persistent rheumatic activity.

However, if the anatomical lesions are suitable for repair, it should be preferred, especially in young patients and women of childbearing age, because of the better long-term event-free survival (fewer thromboembolic and haemorrhagic events) and the fact that lifelong anticoagulant treatment is not required.

For Nobyoschi [139], the 4 patients operated on for post-DMPC MI had an RVM. In the series by Boussada et al [140], 2 patients underwent surgery for traumatic MI. The first had a rupture of the cords of the small mitral valve and underwent RVM, while the second had a tear of the large mitral valve and underwent mitral commissuroplasty.

In the series by Kotsuka [141], all patients with traumatic MI underwent RVM.

In the series by Kaul et al [142], significant mitral regurgitation was observed in 120 patients (3.3% of patients with CPPD), of whom 66 patients required urgent mitral valve replacement and 54 patients received medical treatment. In patients who underwent valve replacement, the traumatic lesions were a tear of a valve leaflet in 48 patients (72.7%), a rupture of cords in 12 patients (18.2%), and a commissural tear in 6 patients (9.1%).

In Howard's series [143], 21 patients out of 280 with DMPC had severe MI. The lesions were as follows: cord rupture in 45% of cases, valve tear in 30% of cases (anterior valve tear in 1 case and posterior valve tear in 5 cases), and excessive commissural opening in 26% of cases. Seventy-one percent of patients required RVM within the first 6 months following the procedure.

In the series by Varma et al [54], all the patients underwent RVM because the commissures were fused, the valves thickened and fibrosed, and the sub-valvular apparatus remodelled; all the more so because the valve tears were large and involved the mitral annulus.

VII- Results of surgical treatment :

1- Early post-operative follow-up

The surgical procedure is often fraught with considerable risk, as it involves patients with pulmonary oedema and low cardiac output. Intensive perioperative care is required. Weaning patients off mechanical ventilation is a particularly delicate operation, and should not be considered too early, but only when ventricular function has stabilised. The operative mortality rate is 5% [144]. In addition to the early complications of valve prostheses and conservative mitral surgery, a flare-up of PAH with right ventricular dysfunction may be noted in the early postoperative period.

2- Long-term monitoring :

The main aim of clinical monitoring of patients with a mechanical valve prosthesis is to maintain a balance between anti-thrombotic protection and the risk of bleeding, by maintaining an INR of between 2.5 and 3.5 for patients with a mitral prosthesis [124].

Doppler echocardiography is the preferred technique for assessing mitral prosthesis dysfunction. In the literature, in cases of rheumatic disease, the long-term results of plasty are not as satisfactory as for other aetiologies. There is a risk of recurrence through progression of the disease. In the case of valve replacement, the late complications are those of valve prostheses.

VIII- Conclusion:

Mitral insufficiency is the most common and most serious complication following percutaneous mitral dilatation. Its mechanism is often a tear in the large mitral valve. Other possible mechanisms are tear of the small mitral valve, excessive opening of the commissures, valve prolapse due to rupture of the pillar or cords, and para-commissural tears.

It is suspected on the basis of per-procedural haemodynamic data and confirmed by ultrasound study. Pre-existing MI of any degree and pulmonary arterial hypertension are predictive factors for this complication. The morphology of the mitral valve and subvalvular apparatus is well correlated with the occurrence of severe mitral insufficiency after percutaneous mitral dilatation. The degree of commissural calcification rather than valvular calcification in general, and the heterogeneity of lesion distribution rather than severity, are strong predictors of severe mitral leakage.

Practical management of this MI depends on the severity of the leak and clinical tolerance.

Post-CPMS traumatic mitral insufficiency appears to be less amenable to valve repair than other MI aetiologies due to major calcifications, reduced leaflet mobility and extensive remodelling of the valvular or sub-valvular tissue, and often requires valve replacement. However, if the anatomical lesions are suitable for repair, this should be preferred, especially in young patients and women of childbearing age, because of the better long-term event-free survival.

Most series in the literature have used mitral valve replacement exclusively. Other series, such as those by Acar [54] and Abid [136], described a few cases of conservative surgery, particularly in cases of paracommissural and leaflet valve tears.

Surgery for acute mitral insufficiency is associated with a high morbidity and mortality rate. The long-term results of plasty are not as satisfactory as for other aetiologies. In fact, progression of rheumatic damage is dreadful. In the case of valve replacement, the late complications are those of valve prostheses.

Bibliography :

[1] Wilkins GT, Weyman AE, Abascal VM, PC Block,IF Placios. Percutaneous balloon dilatation of the mitral valve: an analysis of echocardiographic variables related to outcome and the mechanism of dilatation. Br Heart J 1988 vol 60(4): 299308.

[2] Hunsal Mubarak . The anatomy of full term neonate. Gray's Anatomy 39th edition. Elsevier 2008.

[3] Borsali, H. Nougue, A. Mebazaa. Update of the ASA criteria for C2 scoring of pre-anaesthetic consultations. Annales françaises d'anesthésie et de réanimation, September 2013; Volume 32, Issue 9: 622-3.

[4] Parolari A, Pesce LL, Trezzi M, et al. EuroSCORE performance in valve surgery: a meta-analysis. Ann ThoracSurg, 2010;89: 787-93.

[5] Toumpoulis IK, Anagnostopoulos CE, Toumpoulis SK, DeRose JJ, Swistel DG. EuroSCORE predicts long-term mortality after heart valve surgery. Ann Thorac Surg, 2005; 79: 1902-8.

[6] Chlmers J. Validation of EuroSCORE II in a modern cohort of patients undergoing cardiac surgery.Europeen Journal of Cardiothoracic Surgery,2013; 43(4): 688-94.

[7] Alexandre F., Fabiani JN. Extracorporeal circulation. EMC (Elsevier Masson SAS, Paris), Techniques chirurgicales - Thorax, 2007; 42-513.

[8] Epidemiological bulletin of the Tunisian Ministry of Public Health. Tunisie 2005; 2: 8.

[9] Ruiz C, Zhang H, Gamra H, Allen J, Lau F. Late clinical and echographic follow up after percutaneous balloon dilatation of the mitral valve. Br heart J 1994; 71:4548.

[10] lung B, Cormier B, Ducimetiere . Immediate results of percutaneous mitral commissurotomy. A predictive model on a series of 1514 patients. Circulation 1996; 94 (9): 2124-30.

[11] lung B, Baron G, Butchart EG, Delahaye F ,Barwolf CG,OlfA W et al. A prospective survey of patients with valvular heart disease in Europe: the Euro Heart Survey on valvular heart. J 2003; 24: 1231-1243.

[12] Palacios IF. Farewell to surgical mitral commissurotomy for many patients. Circulation1998: 223-226, Vol 97.

[13] Ben Farhat MB, Ayari M, Maatouk F, Betbout F, Gamra H, Jarrar M et al. Percutaneous balloon versus surgical closed and open mitral commissurotomy: Seven-year follow-up results of a randomized trial Circulation 1998 ; 97 (3): 245250.

[14] Kumar A, Kapoor A, Sinha N, Goel PK, Umeshan CV, Tiwari S et al. Influence of sub valvular pathology on immediate results and follow up events of Inoue Balloon Mitral Valvotomy. International Journal of Cardiology 1998; 67 (3): 201209.

[15] Neumayer U, Schmidt HK, Fassbender D, Mannebach H, Bogunovic N, Horstkotte D. Early (three-month) results of percutaneous mitral valvotomy with the Inoue balloon in 1,123consecutive patients comparing various age groups. Am J Cardiol 2002, 90 (2):190-193.

[16] Song JK, Song JM, Kang DH, Sung-C Y, Duk W P, Seung W L et al. Restenosis and adverse events after successful percutaneous mitral valvuloplasty: immediate post-procedural mitral valve area as an important

prognosticator. Eur Heart J 2009; 30: 1254-1262.

[17] Arora R, Singh KG, Ramachandra MGD. Percutaneous transatrial mitral commissurotomy: Immediate and intermediate results. J Am Coll1994; Vol 23: 1327-1332.

[18] Vahanian A, Baumgartner H, Bax J. Guidelines on the management of valvular heart disease. The Task Force on the Management of Valvular Heart Disease of the European Society of Cardiology.European Heart Journal 2007; 28(2): 230-268.

[19] Orrange S, Kawanishi D, Lopez B, Curry S, Rahimtoola S. Actuarial Outcome after Catheter Balloon Commissurotomy in Patients with Mitral Stenosis. Circulation 1997; 95: 382-9.

[20] Sutaria N, Elder A, Shaw T. Long term outcome of percutaneous mitral balloon valvotomy in patients aged 70 and over. Heart 2000; 83: 433-8.

[21] Liu, T.-J., et al, Percutaneous balloon commissurotomy reduces incidence of ischemic cerebral stroke in patients with symptomatic rheumatic mitral stenosis. International Journal of Cardiology, 2008. 123(2): pp. 189-190.

[22] Ünal S, Narin A. Mitral balloon valvotomy in percutaneous balloon valvotomy. Renk publisher Company-Istambul Turkey.1991: 67 - 121.

[23] Block PC, Palacios JF, Block EH, Tuzcu ME, Griffin B. Late (two year) followup after percutaneous balloon mitral valvotorny. Am. J. Cardiol 1992; 69: 537-541.

[24] Hernandez R, Banuelos C, Alfonso F, Goicolea J, Fernandez-Ortiz A, Escaned J, AzconaL et al. Long-Term Clinical and Echocardiographic Follow-up after Percutaneous Mitral Valvuloplasty with the Inoue Balloon. Circulation 1999; 99:1580-6.

[25] lung B, Garbarz E, Michaud P, Mahdhaoui A, Helou S, Farah B ET al. Percutaneous mitral commissurotomy for restenosis after surgical commissurotomy.The Am coll of card 2000; 35: 1295- 302.

[26] Ben Farhat M, Betbout F, Gamra H, Maatouk F, Ayari M, Cherif A .l. Results of percutaneous Double balloon mitral commissurotomy in one medical center in Tunisia. Am J Card 1995; 76:1266-70.

[27] Pathan AZ, Mahdi NA, Leon MN, Lopez Cuellar J, Simosa H, Block PC et al. Is redo percutaneous mitral balloon valvuloplasty indicated in patients with post- PMV mitral restenosis? J Am CollCardiol 1999; 34:49-54.

[28] lung, A NicoudHouel, O Fondard, H Akoudad, T Haghighat, E Brochet et al. Temporal trends in percutaneous mitral commissurotomy over a 15-year period. Eur Heart J (2004); 25 (8): 701-707.

[29] Vahanian A, Michel PL, Cormier B, Ghanem G, Vitoux B, Maroni JP et al. Immediate and mid-term results of percutaneous mitral commissurotomy. Eur Heart J 1991; 12 (suppl B): 84-9.

[30] Alfonso F ,Macaya C, Hernandez R, Banuelos C, Goicolea J, Iniguez A et al. Early and late results of percutaneous mitral valvuloplasty for mitral stenosis associated with mild mitral regurgitation. Am J Cardiol 1993; 71: 1304-10.

[31] Chen CR, Cheng TO. Percutaneous balloon mitral valvuloplasty by the Inoue technique: a multicenter study of 4832 patients in China.Am Heart J 1995; 129: 1197-203.

[32] Padial R, Freitas N, Sagie A, JB. Newell, AE.Weyman, Robert A et al. Echocardiography can predict which patients will develop severe mitral regurgitation after percutaneous mitral valvulotomy. Journal of the American College of Cardiology1996; 27 (5): 1225-1231.

[33] Cannan CR, RA.Nischumira,GS.Reeder ,DR.Ilstrup,DR.Larson, DR.Holmes et al. Echocardiographic assessment of commissural calcium: a simple predictor of outcome after percutaneous mitral balloon valvotomy. J Am CollCardiol 1997; 29:175-80.

[34] Mueller UK, Sareli P, Essop MR. Anterior mitral leaflet retraction. A new echocardiographic predictor of severe mitral regurgitation following balloon valvuloplasty by the Inoue technique. Am J Cardiol 1998; 81: 656-9.

[35] Chiang CW, Hsu LA, Chu PH, Ko YS, Ko YL, Cheng NJ et al. On-line Multiplane transoesophageal echocardiography for balloon mitral commissurotomy. Am J Cardiol 1998; 515-8.

[36] Padial LR, Abascal VM, Moreno PR, Weyman AE, Levine RA, Palacios IF. Echocardiography can predict the development of severe mitral regurgitation after percutaneous mitral valvuloplasty by the Inoue technique. Am J Cardiol 1999; 83:1210-3.

[37] Kang DH, Park SW, Song JK. Long-term clinical and echocardiographic outcome of percutaneous mitral valvuloplasty. Randomized comparison of Inoue and double-balloon techniques. J Am Coll Cardiol 2000; 35:169-75.

[38] Ben Farhat M. Freedom restenosis after percutaneous double balloon mitral commissurotomy. Am Heart J 2001; 142:1072-9.

[39] Arora R , Kalra GS, Singh S , Mukhopadhyay S, Kumar A , Mohan JC et al.Percutaneoustransvenous mitral commissurotomy: Immediate and long-term follow-up results. Catheterization and Cardiovascular Interventions 2002; 55 (4): 450-456.

[40] Konka M, Chmielak Z, Ruzyllo, Hoffman P, W. How to predict development of severe mitral regurgitation after percutaneous mitral commissurotomy? Przegl Lek 2004:61(6):725-8.

[41] Hani Jneid, Ignacio Cruz-Gonzalez, María Sanchez-Ledesma, Andrew O. Maree, Roberto J. Cubeddu, Milton L. Leon et al mpact of Pre- and Postprocedural Mitral Regurgitation on Outcomes Alter Percutaneous Mitral Valvuloplasty for Mitral Stenosis. Am J Cardiol 2009; 104:1122-1127).

[42] Saaidi Imen, Predictive factors and mechanism of mitral insufficiency after percutaneous mitral dilatation: an echographic study of 150 cases. Thesis of the Faculty of Medicine of Tunis: 2005;TO 235/2005.

[43] Julio C. Echarte M, Juan Valiente M. Severe Mitral Regurgitation After Percutaneous Mitral Valvuloplasty . Rev Argent Cardiol 2010; 78:222-227.

[44] Korkmaz S, Demirkan B, Güray Y, Yilmaz MB, Aksu T, §a§maz H .Acute and long-term follow-up results of percutaneous mitral balloon valvuloplasty: a singlecenter study.Anadolu Kardiyol Derg 2011; 11: 515-20.

[45] Chauvaud S. Plasties mitrales: techniques chirurgicales; EMC techniques chirurgicales 42-532.

[46] Nobuyoshi M, Arita T, Shirai S, Hamasaki N, Yokoi H , Lwabuchi M et al. Percutaneous Balloon Mitral Valvuloplasty: A Review. Circulation 2009, Vol 119: 211-219.

[47] Acar C, Vahanian A, Grare P , Pascal P. Traumatic mitral insufficiency after percutaneous dilatation. Mechanisms and techniques. Arch Mal cœur 1991; 84: 1529-34.

[48] Jneid, H., et al, Impact of pre-and postprocedural mitral regurgitation on outcomes after percutaneous mitral valvuloplasty for mitral stenosis. The American Journal of Cardiology, 2009. 104(8): pp. 1122-1127.

[49] Ritto D, Sutherland GR, Currie P, Starkey IR, Shax TRD. The comparative value of transoesophageal and transthoracic echocardiography before and after percutaneous mitral valvulotomy: a prospective study: Am

Heart J 1993.125:1094110.

[50]   Park SH, Kim MA, Hyon MS. The advantages of on line transoesophagealechogardiography guide during percutaneous balloon valvuloplasty. J Am SocEchocardiogra 200; 13: 26-34

[51]   Predergast BD, Shaw TRD, Lung B, Vahanian A, Northridge DB. Conteporaryciteria for the selection of patients for percutaneous balloon mitral valvuloplasty. Heart 2002; 87: 401-4

[52]   Sutaria N, Northridge DB, Shaw TRD. Significance of commissural calcification on outcome of mitral valvotomy. Heart 2000; 84: 398-402.

[53] Akin M , Sagcan A, Nalbangil S .The predictive value of mitral leaflet motion and thickness index scores on early restonosis after mitral balloon valvuloplasty. Tex Heart Inst J2004; 31: 251-6.

[54] Varma PK1, Theodore S, Neema PK, Ramachandran P, Sivadasanpillai H, Nair KK, Neelakandhan KS. Emergency surgery after percutaneous trans mitral commissurotomy: operative versus echocardiographic findings, mechanisms of complications, and outcomes. J Thoracic Cardio vasc Surg 2005; 130(3):772-6.

[55] Gross RL, Cunningham JN, Snively SL. Long- Term results of open radical mitral commissurotomy: ten year follow -up study of 202 patients. Am J Cardiol 1981; 47:821-5.

[56] Reifart N, Nowak B , Baykut D, Satter P, Bussmann WD, Kaltenbach M. Experimental balloon valvuloplasty of fibrotic and calcific mitral valves. Circulation 1990; 81: 1005-11.

[57] A Cequier, R Bonnan , J Crepeau J,Dethy M,I Dyrda, D Watters.Massive mitral regurgitation caused by tearing of the anterior leaflet during percutaneous mitral balloon valvuloplasty. The American Journal of Medicine; July 1988; volume 85:100-103.

[58] Wei T, Zeng C, Chen F,Wang C,Chen L, Chen Q et al .Influence of commissural calcification on the immediate outcomes of percutaneous

balloon mitral valvuloplasty .ActaCardiol 2003;58:411-5.

[59] Agarwal BL, Kappor A, Singh R. Predective accuracy of commissural pathlogy and its role in determining the outcome following Innoue balloon mitral valvotomy. Indian Heart J2002; 54:39-45.

[60] Zaki AM, Kasem HH, Bakhoum S, Mokhtar M, El Naggar W, White CJ et al. Comparison of early results of percutaneous metallic mitral commissurotome with Inoue balloon technique in patients with high mitral echocardiographic scores. Catheter Cardiovasc Intervent 2002; 57:312-7.

[61] Vahanian A, Michel PL, Cormier B, et al. Results of percutaneous mitral commissurotomy in 200 patients. Am J Cardiol 1989;63:847-52.

[62] Gerosa G1, Fracasso A, Guzzi G, Muneretto C, Thiene G, Casarotto D. Emergency surgical treatment of ruptured incompetent mitral valve after percutaneous valvuloplasty. J Heart Valve Dis. 1993 Sep; 2(5):523-8.

[63] Chern MS, Chang HJ, Lin FC, Wu D. String-plucking as a mechanism of chordal rupture during balloon mitral valvuloplasty using Inoue balloon catheter. Catheter Cardiovasc Interv. 1999; 47: 213-7.

[64] Carrillo X, Lopez-Ayerbe J, Ferrer E, Ruyra X. Mitral Valve Repair Surgery for Traumatic Rupture of the Anterolateral Papillary Muscle-Letters to the Editor. RevEsp Cardiol. 2008; 61(12):1355-65 .

[65] Acar C1, Jebara VA, Grare P, Chachques JC, Dervanian P, Vahanian A et al. Traumatic mitral insufficiency following percutaneous mitral dilation: anatomic lesions and surgical implications. Eur J Cardiothorac Surg. 1992; 6(12):660-3; discussion 663-4.

[66] Gopalakrishnan A, Ganapathi S, Sivasubramonian S, Sivadasanpillai H. Partial papillary muscle rupture following percutaneous mitral valvuloplasty without mitral regurgitation. J Echocardiogr. 2016 ; 47: 213-7.

[67] Demirkol S, Unlu M, Balta S, Yuksel UC, Celik T. Mitral antrolataral papillary muscle rupture in an asymptomatic patient with mitral stenosis

after percutaneous mitral balloon valvuloplasty. Echocardiography 2012 Oct: 29(9):E250.

[68] Acar G,Toprak C, Avci A, Afe SC, Esen AM. Posteromedial papillary muscle rupture following percutaneous mitral balloon vavotomy. Echocardiography 2014 May: 31(5): E156-7.

[69] Giovanni Domenico Cresce, Alessandro Favaro , Augusto D'Onofrio,, Caterina Piccin, Paolo Magagna, Massimo Spanghero et al. Post-Traumatic Rupture of the Anterolateral Papillary Muscle. Ann Thorac Surg 2009; 88: 1664-6.

[70] Kaul UA, Singh S, Kalra GS, Nair M, Mohan JC, Nigam M, et al. Mitral regurgitation following percutaneous transvenous mitral commissurotomy. J Heart Valve Dis. 2000; 9: 262-6.

[71] Kaul, U., et al, Mitral regurgitation following percutaneous transvenous mitral commissurotomy: a single-center experience. The Journal of Heart Valve Disease, 2000. 9(2): pp. 262-266, discussion 266-268.

[72] Varma PK1, Theodore S, Neema PK, Ramachandran P, Sivadasanpillai H, Nair KK et al.
Emergency surgery after percutaneous transmitral commissurotomy: operative versus echocardiographic findings, mechanisms of complications, and outcomes. J Thorac Cardiovasc Surg. 2005 Sep; 130(3):772-6.

[73] Bonow RO, Carabello B, De Leon AC, et al. ACC/AHA Guidelines for the management of patients with valvular heart disease. A report of the American College of Cardiology/American Heart Association Task Force on Practice Guidelines. J Am CollCardiol 2006; 48:e1- 148.

[74] Nobuyoshi M1, Hamasaki N, Kimura T, Nosaka H, Yokoi H, Yasumoto H, et al. Indications, complicationsand short-term clinical outcome of percutaneous transvenous mitral commissurotomy. Circulation

1989; 80: 782-92.

[75] Herrmann HC, Ramaswamy K, Isner JM, Kaskuf R . Factors influencing immediate results, complications and short-term follow-up status after inoue balloon mitral valvotomy: a North American multicenter study.Am Heart J 1992 ;124: 1606.

[76] Cohen DJ, Kuntz RE, Gordon SP. Predictors of long-term outcome after percutaneous balloon mitral valvuloplasty. N Engl J Med 1992; 327:1329 -1331.

[77] Palacios IF. Techniques of balloon valvotomy for mitral stenosis. In:Robicsk F, editor. Cardiac Surgery. State of the Art Reviews, vol. 5.Philadelphia: Hanley and Belfus, 1991: 229 -38.

[78] Zhang L, Wei W, Yue XY, Shi ZG. The impact of mitral valve morphology on the short and long-term outcome post percutaneous balloon mitral valvuloplasty in patients with mitral valve stenosis.ZhonghuaXinXue Guan Bing ZaZhi. 2011 Dec; 39 (12):1124-8.

[79] Garcia-CastilloA, TrevinoA. J, Ibarra M .Mitral insufficiency after mitral balloon-catheter valvuloplasty: its incidence,predictive factors and prognosis. Archivos de lInstituto de Cardiologiade Mexico1995; 65, no1, p: 39-47.

[80] The national Heart, Lung and Blood Institute Balloon Valvuloplasty Registry Participants. Multicenter experience with balloon mitral commissurotomy: the NHLBI balloon valvuloplasty registry report on immediate and 30-day follow-up results. Circulation 1992; 85: 448-61

[81] Feldman T, Caroll JD, Isner JM. Effect of valve deformity on results and mitral regurgitation after Inoue balloon commissurotomy. Circulation 1992; 85: 180-7.

[82] Mattos C, Braga SLN, Esteves CA. Percutaneous mitral valvotomy in patients eighteen years old and younger. Immediate and late results. Arq Bras Cardiol 1999; 73: 378-81.

[83] Reid CL, Chandraratna PAN, Kawanishi DT, Kotlewski A, RahimtoolaSH. Influence of mitral valve morphology on double-balloon catheter balloon valvuloplasty in patients with mitral stenosis. Analysis of factors predicting immediate and 3-month results. Circulation 1989; 80: 515-24.

[84] Krassuski RA,Warner JJ,Peterson G.Comparison of results of percutaneous balloon mitral commissurotomy in patients aged > 65 years with those in patients aged < 65 years.Am J Cardiol 2001;88:994-1000.

[85] Hung JS, Cherm MS, Wu JJ, Morgan Fu, Kou-Ho Yen, Yahn-Chyurn Wu et al. Short and long results of catheter balloon percutaneous

[86] Iung B, Cormier B, Berdah P, et al. Is it possible to predict severe mitral regurgitation following percutaneous mitral commissurotomy? Test of a multivariate model on 1514 cases. Circulation 1997; 96(suppl I): 204.

[87] Garbarz E, Iung B, Cormier B, Vahanian A. Echocardiographic criteria in selection of patients for percutaneous mitral commissurotomy. Echocardiogaphy 1999; 16: 711-21.

[88] Lau KW, Hung JS. Balloon impasse: a marker for severe mitral subvalvular disease and a predictor of mitral regurgitation in Inoue balloon percutaneous transvenous mitral commissurotomy. Cathet Cardiovasc Diagn 1995; 35:310-9.

[89] Chen C, Wang X, Wang Y. Value of two-dimensional echocardiography in selecting patients and balloon sizes for percutaneous balloon mitral valvuloplasty. J Am CollCardiol 1989; 14: 1651-8.

[90] Rifaie O, Esmat I, AbdelrahmenM . Can a novel Echocardiographic Score Better Predict outcome after Percutaneous Balloon Mitral Valvuloplasty? Echocardiography 2009; 26: 119-127.

[91] Bezdah L, Drissa MA, Ksari R, Baccar H, Belhani H.,Echocardiographic parameters predictive of immediate outcome of percutaneous mitral commissurotomy. La Tunisie Médicale 2007; 85: 479-

484.

[92] Gross RI, Cunningham JN, Snively SL, et al. Long-term results of open radical mitral commissurotomy: ten year follow-up study of 202 patients. Am J Cardiol 1981; 47: 821-5.

[93] Sanati, H., et al, Mitral valve resistance determines hemodynamic consequences of severe rheumatic mitral stenosis and immediate outcomes of percutaneous valvuloplasty. Echocardiography. 2017;34:162-168.

[94] Reifart N, Nowak B, Baykut D, Satter P, Bussmann WD, Kaltenbach M. Experimental balloon valvuloplasty of fibrotic and calcific mitral valves. Circulation 1990; 81: 1005-11.

[95] Maaoqin S, Guoxiang H, Zhiyuan S, Luxiang C, Houyuan H, Liangyi S, et al. The clinical and hemodynamic results of mitral balloon valvuloplasty for patients with mitral stenosis complicated by severe pulmonary hypertension. Eur J Intern Med 2005Oct; 16(6): 413-8.

[96] Wisenbaugh T, Essop R, Middlemost S, Skoularigis J, Rothlisberger C, Skudicky D, et al. Effects of severe pulmonary hypertension on outcome of balloon mitral valvotomy. Am J Cardiol 1992 vol 70: 823-5.

[97] S Pande, Surendra K. Agarwal, Aditya Kapoor, Sudeep Kumar. Implications of Left Atrial Size in Rheumatic Mitral Valve Disease Undergoing Mitral Valve Replacement. Heart, Lung and Circulation, Volume 20, Issue 12, December 2011, Pages 801-802.

[98] Hildick-Smith D J R, ShapiroLM. Balloon mitral valvuloplasty in the elderly. Eur Heart J 2000; 83: 374-375.

[99] Palacios IF, Sanchez PL, Harell LC, Weyman AE, Block PC.Which patients benefit from percutaneous mitral balloon valvuloplasty? Pre valvuloplasty and post valvuloplasty variables that predict long-term outcome. Circulation 2002; 105: 146571.

[100] Ignacio Cruz-Gonzalez, Maria Sanchez-Ledesma, Pedro L. Sanchez. Predicting Success And Long-Term Outcomes Of Percutaneous

Mitral Valvuloplasty: A Multifactorial Score. The American Journal Of Medicine (2009).

[102] T. Mailer, R. Petitclerc, J. Lesperance . Mitral regurgitation assessed by echoDoppler after percutaneous mitral valvuloplasty. Circulation, vol. 80, no. 2, supplement II, p16 (Abstract) 1989.

[103] Sancho M, Medina A ,Suarez J, Hernandez E, Pan M, Coello I et al. Factors influencing progression of mitral regurgitation after transarterial balloon valvuloplasty for mitral stenosis.Am J Cardiol 1990;66:737-40.

[104] Cormier B, Vahanian A, Micel PL et al. Two-dimensional ultrasound and Doppler evaluation of the results of percutaneous mitral valvuloplasty. Arch Mal Cœur 1989; 82: 185-91.

[105] Nobuyoschi, Hamasaki , Kimura T, Nasaka H , InouéK. Indications , complications and short term clinical outcome of percutaneous transvenous mitral commissurotomy. Circulation 1989;80:782-92 .

[106] Abascal VM, Wilkins GT, Choong CY, Block PC, Palacios IF, Weyman AE. Mitral regurgttation after percutaneous balloon mitral valvuloplasty in adults Evaluation by pulsed Doppler echocardiogram.J Am Co Cardiol 1988: I1:257-263.

[107] McKay RG, Kawanishi DT, Rahimtoola SH. Catheter balloon valvuloplasty of the mitral valve in adults using a double-balloon technique. Early hemcdynamic results. JAMA 1987:257:1753-1761.

[108] Chen CR, Lo ZX, Hung ZD, Inoue KJ, Cheng TO. The Chinese experience in 30 patients. Am Hearf J cardiovascSurg 19X4:87:39-402. 1988; 115:937-947.

[109] Seung-Jung Park, MD, Jae-Joong Kim, MD, Seong-Wook Park, MD, Jae- Kwan Song, MD, Phil,Young-Cheoul Doo, MD, and Simon Jong-Koo Lee, MD. Immediate and one year results of mitral balloon valvuloplasty using Inoue and doube balloon-techniques. Am J cardiol 1993; 71-938943.

[110] HermannH.C, Feldman T, Isner J.M, Bashore T, Holmes D.R, RothBaum D.A et al. Comparison of results of percutaneous balloon valvuloplasty in patients with mild and moderate mitral stenosis to those with severe mitral stenosis. Am. J. Cardiol 1993; 71: 1300-1303.

[111] Inoue K., Hung J.S. Percutaneous transvenous mitral commissurotomy (PTMC): the far east experience. Text book of Interventional Cardiology Edited by TopolE.l. W.B. Saunders Company Philadelphia 1990 pp 887-895.

[112] Zaibag MA, Alkasab, Ribero PA , Alfagih MR.Percutaneous double balloon mitral valvulotomy for rheumatic mitral valve stenosis.Lance,1986;8484: 757-766.

[113] Jui-Sung Hung, Kean-Wah Lau, Ping-Han Lo, Ming-Shyan Chern, Jong-Jen Wu.Complications of Inoue balloon mitral commissurotomy: Impact of operator experience and evolving technique. Am Heart J 1999; 138:114-21.

[114] Hernandez R,Macaya C,Banuelos C,Alfonso A,Goicolea J,IniGuez A et al.Predictors , Mechnisms and outcome of severe mitral regurgitation complicating percutaneous mitral valvotomy with the Inoue Balloon. Am J Cardiol 1992; 70:11691174.

[115] Tucuzu M, Block P,Palacios IF. Comparison of early versus late experience with percutaneous mitral balloon valvulotomy. Am J Cardiol 1991; 17:1121-1124.

[116] Golbasi Z, Ucar O, Keles T. Increased levels of high sensitive C-reactive protein in patients with chronic rheumatic valve disease: evidence of ongoing inflammation. Eur J Heart Fail 2002; 4:593 - 5.

[117] S. Harikrishnan , E. Rajeev, Jaganmohan A. Tharakan .Acute phase reactants predict mitral regurgitation following mitral valvuloplasty. International journal of cardiology; 112 (2006) 127.

[118] Hung JS, Chern MS, Wu JJ, Fu M, Yeh KH, Wu YC et al. Short and

long-term results of catheter balloon percutaneous transvenous mitral commissurotomy. Am J Cardiol 1991; 67: 854-62.

[119] Greutmann Met Silversides CK. The ROPAC registry: a multicentre collaboration on pregnancy outcomes in women with heart disease. Eur Heart J.2013; 34: 634-5.

[120] Borna S, Borna H and Hantooshzadeh S. Pregnancy outcomes in women with heart disease. Int J Gynecol Obstet.2006; 92:122-23.

[121] Gamra H, Ben-Farhat M, Betbout F et al. Long term outcome of balloon mitral commissurotomy during pregnancy: A prospective physical and mental evaluation of babies. Euro Interv.2006; 2:302-9

[122] Ben Farhat M, Gamra H, Betbout Fet al. Percutaneous balloon mitral commissurotomy during pregnancy. Heart.1997; 77:564-7.

[123] Gupta A, Lokhandwala Y, Satoskar P et al. Balloon Mitral Valvotomy in Pregnancy: Maternal and Fetal Outcomes. J Am Coll Surg.1998; 187:409-15.

43.

[124] Esteves C, S. Munoz J, Braga S et al. Immediate and Long-Term Follow-Up of Percutaneous Balloon Mitral Valvuloplasty in Pregnant Patients With Rheumatic Mitral Stenosis. Am J Cardiol.2006; 98 :812-816.

[125] Grewal KS, Malkowski MJ, Pirasha AR et al. Effect of general anesthesia on the severity of mitral regurgitation by transeosophageal echocardiography. Am J Cardiol 2000; 85: 199-203.

[126] Lei Q, Wei X, Huang K, Xie B. Lacerated anterior mitral valve leaflet following percutaneous balloon valvuloplasty, J Card Surg, 2017, 28-29.

[127] Nishimura et al. 2014/ACC Guideline for the Management of Patients With Valvular Heart Disease Journal of the American College of Cardiology 2014 by the American Heart Association, Inc, and the American College of Cardiology Foundation Published by Elsevier Inc.

[128] Alec Vahanian. Guidelines on the management of valvular heart disease. European Heart Journal, 2012; 33: 2451-96.

[129] Bayya PR, Varma PK, Raman SP, Neema PK. Emergency mitral valve replacement for acute severe mitral regurgitation following balloon mitral valvotomy: Pathophysiology of hemodynamic collapse and peri-operative management issues.

[130] Price LC, Wort SJ, Finney SJ, Marino PS, Brett SJ. Pulmonary vascular and right ventricular dysfunction in adult critical care: Current and emerging options for management: A systematic literature review. Crit Care 2010; 14: R169.

[131] Gerhardt MA, Booth JV, Chesnut LC et al. Acute myocardial beta-adrenergic receptor dysfunction after cardiopulmonary bypass in patients with cardiac valve disease. Circulation 1998; 98: II275-II281.

[132] Chassot PG,Bettex D. Précis of cardiac anaesthesia 2011: Chapter 11.

[133] S. Chauvaud. Surgery for acquired mitral valve lesions: generalities. EMC - Techniques chirurgicales-Thorax 2011:1-6 [Article 42-530].

[134] Gewal KS, Mallowski MJ, Pirascha et al. Effect of general anesthesia in on the severity of mitral regurgitation by transosophageal echocardiography.Am J Cardiol 2000; 85:199-203.

[135] Jong-Won Ha, Namsik Chung, Byung-Chul Chang, Yangsoo Jang, Won- Heum Shim, Seung-Yun Cho and Sung-Soon Kim.Acute Mitral Regurgitation Due to Leaflet Tear After Balloon Valvotomy. Circulation 1998; 98:2095-2097.

[136] Abid Noomen. Les accidents chirurgicaux de la dilatation mitrale percutanée. Doctoral thesis in medicine 1994; Faculty of Medicine, Tunis.

[137] Chauvaud S. EMC-Techniques chirurgicales thorax 2012 Volume 42 ; 532.

[138] Gonçalo F. Coutinho, Carlos Filipe Branco, Elisabete Jorge, Pedro

M. Correia, Manuel J. Antunes.Mitral Valve Surgery after percutaneous mitral valvuloplasty.Is repair still feasible. European Journal of Cardio-Thoracic Surgery 47 (2015): 1-6.

[139] Nubyyoschi, Hamsaki N, Kimura T, Nasaka H, Inoué K. Indications, complications and short term clinical outcome of percutaneous tranvenous mitral commissurotomy. Circulation 1989; 80: 782-92.

[140] Boussada R. Percutaneous mitral balloon commissurotomy in mitral stenosis: immediate and medium-term results .thèse de médecine Tunis 1990.

[141] Kotsuka Y1, Furuse A, Yagyu K, Kawauchi M, Takeda M, Hirata K. Mitral valve replacement after percutaneous transvenous mitral commissurotomy. Cardiovasc Surg. 1996 Aug; 4 (4): 530-5.

[142] Kaul UA, Singh S, Kalra GS, Nair M, Mohan JC, Nigam M et al :Mitral regurgitation following percutaneous transvenous mitral commissurotomy: a singlecenter experience. J Heart Valve Dis. 2000 Mar; 9(2):262-6; discussion 266-8.

[143] Howard C.Hermann MD, Joao A.C. Lima, Ted Feldman, Robert Chisholm, Jeffrey Isner, William O'Neill et al. Mechanisms ad outcome of mitral regurgitation after Inoue balloon valvuloplasty.JAC vo l22 N°3 . September 1993;783-9.

[144] Akins CW, Miller DC, Turina MI, Kouchoukos NT, Blackstone EH, Grunkemeier GL et al. Guidelines for reporting mortality and morbidity after cardiac valve interventions. Eur J Cardiothorac Surg 2008; 33: 523-8.

Table of Contents

I-   Introduction 2

II-   Epidemiological characteristics of patients 4

III-   Immediate results of the procedure 5

Bibliography 44

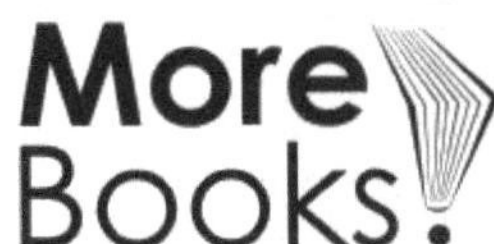

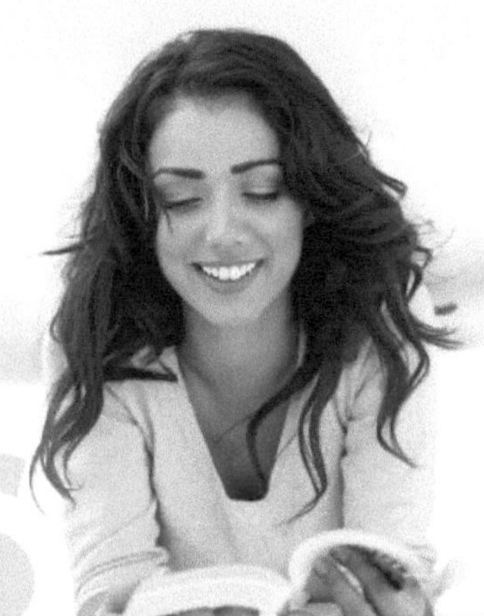

yes
I want morebooks!

Buy your books fast and straightforward online - at one of world's fastest growing online book stores! Environmentally sound due to Print-on-Demand technologies.

Buy your books online at
www.morebooks.shop

Kaufen Sie Ihre Bücher schnell und unkompliziert online – auf einer der am schnellsten wachsenden Buchhandelsplattformen weltweit! Dank Print-On-Demand umwelt- und ressourcenschonend produzi ert.

Bücher schneller online kaufen
www.morebooks.shop

info@omniscriptum.com
www.omniscriptum.com

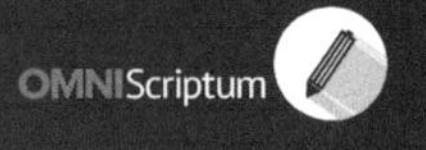

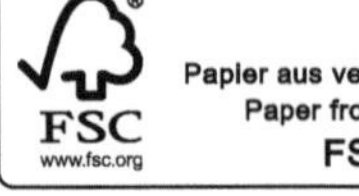

Printed by Books on Demand GmbH, Norderstedt / Germany